ELUSIVE ANTIDOTES: PROGRESS DEVELOPING CHEMICAL, BIOLOGICAL, RADIOLOGICAL AND NUCLEAR COUNTERMEASURES

HEARING

BEFORE THE

SUBCOMMITTEE ON NATIONAL SECURITY, EMERGING THREATS, AND INTERNATIONAL RELATIONS

OF THE

COMMITTEE ON GOVERNMENT REFORM

HOUSE OF REPRESENTATIVES

ONE HUNDRED NINTH CONGRESS

FIRST SESSION

JUNE 14, 2005

Serial No. 109–83

Printed for the use of the Committee on Government Reform

Available via the World Wide Web: http://www.gpoaccess.gov/congress/index.html
http://www.house.gov/reform

U.S. GOVERNMENT PRINTING OFFICE

24–084 PDF   WASHINGTON : 2005

COMMITTEE ON GOVERNMENT REFORM

TOM DAVIS, Virginia, *Chairman*

CHRISTOPHER SHAYS, Connecticut
DAN BURTON, Indiana
ILEANA ROS-LEHTINEN, Florida
JOHN M. McHUGH, New York
JOHN L. MICA, Florida
GIL GUTKNECHT, Minnesota
MARK E. SOUDER, Indiana
STEVEN C. LaTOURETTE, Ohio
TODD RUSSELL PLATTS, Pennsylvania
CHRIS CANNON, Utah
JOHN J. DUNCAN, Jr., Tennessee
CANDICE S. MILLER, Michigan
MICHAEL R. TURNER, Ohio
DARRELL E. ISSA, California
GINNY BROWN-WAITE, Florida
JON C. PORTER, Nevada
KENNY MARCHANT, Texas
LYNN A. WESTMORELAND, Georgia
PATRICK T. McHENRY, North Carolina
CHARLES W. DENT, Pennsylvania
VIRGINIA FOXX, North Carolina

HENRY A. WAXMAN, California
TOM LANTOS, California
MAJOR R. OWENS, New York
EDOLPHUS TOWNS, New York
PAUL E. KANJORSKI, Pennsylvania
CAROLYN B. MALONEY, New York
ELIJAH E. CUMMINGS, Maryland
DENNIS J. KUCINICH, Ohio
DANNY K. DAVIS, Illinois
WM. LACY CLAY, Missouri
DIANE E. WATSON, California
STEPHEN F. LYNCH, Massachusetts
CHRIS VAN HOLLEN, Maryland
LINDA T. SANCHEZ, California
C.A. DUTCH RUPPERSBERGER, Maryland
BRIAN HIGGINS, New York
ELEANOR HOLMES NORTON, District of
 Columbia

———

BERNARD SANDERS, Vermont
(Independent)

MELISSA WOJCIAK, *Staff Director*
DAVID MARIN, *Deputy Staff Director / Communications Director*
ROB BORDEN, *Parliamentarian*
TERESA AUSTIN, *Chief Clerk*
PHIL BARNETT, *Minority Chief of Staff / Chief Counsel*

SUBCOMMITTEE ON NATIONAL SECURITY, EMERGING THREATS, AND INTERNATIONAL RELATIONS

CHRISTOPHER SHAYS, Connecticut, *Chairman*

KENNY MARCHANT, Texas
DAN BURTON, Indiana
ILEANA ROS-LEHTINEN, Florida
JOHN M. McHUGH, New York
STEVEN C. LaTOURETTE, Ohio
TODD RUSSELL PLATTS, Pennsylvania
JOHN J. DUNCAN, Jr., Tennessee
MICHAEL R. TURNER, Ohio
JON C. PORTER, Nevada
CHARLES W. DENT, Pennsylvania

DENNIS J. KUCINICH, Ohio
TOM LANTOS, California
BERNARD SANDERS, Vermont
CAROLYN B. MALONEY, New York
CHRIS VAN HOLLEN, Maryland
LINDA T. SANCHEZ, California
C.A. DUTCH RUPPERSBERGER, Maryland
STEPHEN F. LYNCH, Massachusetts
BRIAN HIGGINS, New York

EX OFFICIO

TOM DAVIS, Virginia

HENRY A. WAXMAN, California

LAWRENCE J. HALLORAN, *Staff Director and Counsel*
KRISTINE FIORENTINO, *Professional Staff Member*
ROBERT A. BRIGGS, *Clerk*
ANDREW SU, *Minority Professional Staff Member*

CONTENTS

ELUSIVE ANTIDOTES: PROGRESS DEVELOP-
ING CHEMICAL, BIOLOGICAL, RADIOLOGI-
CAL AND NUCLEAR COUNTERMEASURES

TUESDAY, JUNE 14, 2005

HOUSE OF REPRESENTATIVES,
SUBCOMMITTEE ON NATIONAL SECURITY, EMERGING
THREATS, AND INTERNATIONAL RELATIONS,
COMMITTEE ON GOVERNMENT REFORM,
Washington, DC.

The subcommittee met, pursuant to notice, at 2:06 p.m., in room 2154, Rayburn House Office Building, Hon. Christopher Shays (chairman of the subcommittee) presiding.

Present: Representatives: Shays, Marchant, Platts, Duncan, Turner, Kucinich, Van Hollen, Ruppersberger, and Higgins.

Staff present: Lawrence Halloran, staff director and counsel; Kristine Fiorentino, professional staff member; Robert A. Briggs, clerk and professional staff member; Andrew Su, minority professional staff member; and Jean Gosa, minority assistant clerk.

Mr. SHAYS. The Subcommittee on National Security, Emerging Threats, and International Relations' hearing entitled, "Elusive Antidotes: Progress Developing Chemical, Biological, Radiological and Nuclear Countermeasures," is called to order.

First, let me apologize for keeping you waiting. It is not my practice to keep any of you waiting, you have very important things to do.

More than a decade after U.S. armed forces faced exposure to Saddam's chemical arsenal and 4 years after the anthrax attacks here at home, the development of medical countermeasures against unconventional weapons remains an elusive goal. A multitude of Federal offices and programs pursue separate, shifting, often competing priorities without disciplined linkage to a strategy to address the most pressing threats.

By one count last year, 75 high level Federal officials in seven Cabinet departments were responsible for biodefense policies, program execution or budgets. The Department of Health and Human Services, the Department of Homeland Security, the Department of Defense, the Department of Agriculture, the Department of Commerce, the Department of State and the Environmental Protection Agency all have some responsibility for the Nation's defenses against chemical, biological, radiological assaults.

To date, this littered landscape has not been fertile soil for the growth of needed countermeasures against the threats posed by the pathogens, toxins, chemicals and isotopes known to be within the grasp of terrorists. Five years ago, the Defense Science Board saw the need for 57 vaccines, drugs and diagnostics to meet the threat. Today, we have just two of those in hand, both based on old technologies.

The Department of Defense specifically, the Joint Vaccine Acquisition Program, offers a sadly illustrative example of the difficulties plaguing the broader Federal effort. A 2004 study by the Institute of Medicine found the DOD biodefense program fragmented and often prey to competing priorities. Launched in 1997 with $322 million, the JVAP has spent that much and more. Yet lists of JVAP "accomplishments" provided to the subcommittee include just one recently licensed therapeutic, no completed vaccines and two target vaccine programs terminated after significant expenditures.

Without question, countermeasure development is an expensive, technically challenging process that cannot be forced to yield results on an arbitrary timetable. The current approach lacks cohesiveness and urgency. Those trying to advance medical countermeasures face a torturous labyrinth of Federal fiefdoms into which billions disappear, yet very few antidotes have yet to emerge.

In October 2001, this subcommittee held a field hearing on the development of medical countermeasures against biological warfare agents. We met across the street in the Department of Health and Human Services headquarters building, because the Capitol complex was closed for anthrax testing and remediation. We were told aggressive steps were being taken to defend both civilian and military personnel against anthrax, smallpox, botulinum toxin and other likely threats.

Today we find the biodefense pipeline still producing little more than promises of cures to come. Project BioShield represents an essential mechanism to streamline the countermeasure development end game, acquisition, but it can do little to accelerate the glacial process of moving vaccines, drugs and other therapies from basic research to final formulation and licensure. That is a function of leadership, coordination and strict adherence to a threat-based strategy.

We asked our witnesses to describe how greater focus and momentum can be brought to this complex process. They bring world class credentials and unmatched experience to our discussion and we look forward to their testimony and we thank them for their presence here today.

At this time, the Chair would recognize Mr. Marchant.

[The prepared statement of Hon. Christopher Shays follows:]

TOM DAVIS, VIRGINIA,
CHAIRMAN

CHRISTOPHER SHAYS, CONNECTICUT
DAN BURTON, INDIANA
ILEANA ROS-LEHTINEN, FLORIDA
JOHN M. McHUGH, NEW YORK
JOHN L. MICA, FLORIDA
GIL GUTKNECHT, MINNESOTA
MARK E. SOUDER, INDIANA
STEVEN C. LATOURETTE, OHIO
TODD RUSSELL PLATTS, PENNSYLVANIA
CHRIS CANNON, UTAH
JOHN J. DUNCAN, JR., TENNESSEE
CANDICE MILLER, MICHIGAN
MICHAEL R. TURNER, OHIO
DARRELL ISSA, CALIFORNIA
VIRGINIA BROWN-WAITE, FLORIDA
JON C. PORTER, NEVADA
KENNY MARCHANT, TEXAS
LYNN A. WESTMORELAND, GEORGIA
PATRICK T. McHENRY, NORTH CAROLINA
CHARLES W. DENT, PENNSYLVANIA
VIRGINIA FOXX, NORTH CAROLINA

ONE HUNDRED NINTH CONGRESS

Congress of the United States

House of Representatives

COMMITTEE ON GOVERNMENT REFORM

2157 RAYBURN HOUSE OFFICE BUILDING

WASHINGTON, DC 20515–6143

MAJORITY (202) 225–5074
FACSIMILE (202) 225–3974
MINORITY (202) 225–5051
TTY (202) 225–6852

http://reform.house.gov

HENRY A. WAXMAN, CALIFORNIA,
RANKING MINORITY MEMBER

TOM LANTOS, CALIFORNIA
MAJOR R. OWENS, NEW YORK
EDOLPHUS TOWNS, NEW YORK
PAUL E. KANJORSKI, PENNSYLVANIA
CAROLYN B. MALONEY, NEW YORK
ELIJAH E. CUMMINGS, MARYLAND
DENNIS J. KUCINICH, OHIO
DANNY K. DAVIS, ILLINOIS
WM. LACY CLAY, MISSOURI
DIANE E. WATSON, CALIFORNIA
STEPHEN F. LYNCH, MASSACHUSETTS
CHRIS VAN HOLLEN, MARYLAND
LINDA T. SANCHEZ, CALIFORNIA
C.A. DUTCH RUPPERSBERGER,
MARYLAND
BRIAN HIGGINS, NEW YORK
ELEANOR HOLMES NORTON,
DISTRICT OF COLUMBIA

BERNARD SANDERS, VERMONT,
INDEPENDENT

SUBCOMMITTEE ON NATIONAL SECURITY, EMERGING THREATS,
AND INTERNATIONAL RELATIONS
Christopher Shays, Connecticut
Chairman
Room B-372 Rayburn Building
Washington, D.C. 20515
Tel: 202 225-2548
Fax: 202 225-2382

Statement of Rep. Christopher Shays
June 14, 2005

More than a decade after U.S. armed forces faced exposure to Saddam's chemical arsenal, and four years after the anthrax attacks here at home, the development of medical countermeasures against unconventional weapons remains an elusive goal. A multitude of federal offices and programs pursue separate, shifting, often competing priorities without disciplined linkage to a strategy to address the most pressing threats.

By one count last year, seventy-five high-level federal officials in seven Cabinet departments were responsible for biodefense policies, program execution or budgets. The Department of Health and Human Services, the Department of Homeland Security, the Department of Defense, the Department of Agriculture, the Department of Commerce, the Department of State and the Environmental Protection Agency all have some responsibility for the nation's defenses against chemical, biological and radiological assaults.

To date, this littered landscape has not been fertile soil for the growth of needed countermeasures against the threats posed by the pathogens, toxins, chemicals and isotopes known to be within the grasp of terrorists. Five years ago, the Defense Science Board saw the need for fifty-seven vaccines, drugs and diagnostics to meet the threat. Today we have just two of those in hand.

Page 1 of 2

The Department of Defense (DOD), specifically the Joint Vaccine Acquisition Program (JVAP), offers a sadly illustrative example of the difficulties plaguing the broader federal effort. A 2004 study by the Institute of Medicine (IOM) found the DOD biodefense program fragmented and often prey to competing priorities. Launched in 1997 with $322 million, the JVAP has spent that much, and more. Yet lists of JVAP "accomplishments" provided to the Subcommittee include just one recently licensed therapeutic, no completed vaccines and two target vaccine programs terminated after significant expenditures.

Without question, countermeasure development is an expensive, technically challenging process that cannot be forced to yield results on an arbitrary timetable. But the current approach lacks cohesiveness and urgency. Those trying to advance medical countermeasures face a torturous labyrinth of federal fiefdoms into which billions disappear. Very few antidotes have yet to emerge.

In October 2001, this Subcommittee held a "field" hearing on the development of medical countermeasures against biological warfare agents. We met across the street, in the Department of Health and Human Services headquarters building, because the Capitol complex was closed for anthrax testing and remediation. We were told aggressive steps were being taken to defend both civilian and military personnel against anthrax, smallpox, botulinum toxin and other likely threats.

But today we find the biodefense pipeline still producing little more than promises of cures to come. Project BioShield represents an essential mechanism to streamline the countermeasure development endgame – acquisition. But it does little to accelerate the glacial process of moving vaccines, drugs and other therapies from basic research to final formulation and licensure. That is a function of leadership, coordination and strict adherence to a threat-based strategy.

We asked our witnesses to describe how greater focus and momentum can be brought to this complex process. They bring world class credentials and unmatched experience to our discussion, and we look forward to their testimony.

Mr. MARCHANT. I don't have any opening statement. I am happy to be here.

Mr. SHAYS. Thank you. I appreciate the gentleman's participation and his help with the work of this subcommittee.

Let me now take care of some business. I ask unanimous consent, given that we have a quorum, that all members of the subcommittee be permitted to place an opening statement in the record and the record remain open for 3 days for that purpose. Without objection, so ordered.

I ask further unanimous consent that all witnesses be permitted to include their written statements in the record and without objection, so ordered.

At this time, I will introduce the first panel. We have Dr. Dale Klein, Assistant to the Secretary of Defense for Nuclear, Chemical and Biological Defense Programs, Department of Defense; Dr. Anthony S. Fauci, Director, National Institute of Allergy and Infectious Diseases, National Institute of Health; the Honorable Stewart Simonson, Assistant Secretary for Public Health, Emergency Preparedness, Department of Health and Human Services; Dr. John Vitko, Jr., Director, Biological Countermeasures Portfolio, Science and Technology Directorate, Department of Homeland Security; and Dr. Ronald J. Saldarini, Scientific Consultant, Institute of Medicine.

As is the custom, we swear our witnesses and I would ask you to stand.

[Witnesses sworn.]

Mr. SHAYS. We prefer that your testimony be closer to 5 minutes but we will roll it over for another 5 minutes and would like you to stop within that time because we have a number of panelists.

Dr. Klein.

STATEMENTS OF DALE KLEIN, ASSISTANT TO THE SECRETARY OF DEFENSE FOR NUCLEAR, CHEMICAL AND BIOLOGICAL DEFENSE PROGRAMS, DEPARTMENT OF DEFENSE; DR. ANTHONY S. FAUCI, DIRECTOR, NATIONAL INSTITUTE OF ALLERGY AND INFECTIOUS DISEASES, NATIONAL INSTITUTE OF HEALTH; STEWART SIMONSON, ASSISTANT SECRETARY FOR PUBLIC HEALTH, EMERGENCY PREPAREDNESS, DEPARTMENT OF HEALTH AND HUMAN SERVICES; JOHN VITKO, JR., DIRECTOR, BIOLOGICAL COUNTERMEASURES PORTFOLIO, SCIENCE AND TECHNOLOGY DIRECTORATE, DEPARTMENT OF HOMELAND SECURITY; AND RONALD J. SALDARINI, SCIENTIFIC CONSULTANT, INSTITUTE OF MEDICINE

STATEMENT OF DALE KLEIN

Dr. KLEIN. Chairman Shays and members of the subcommittee, I am honored to appear before your subcommittee again to address your questions regarding the Department's efforts to develop and acquire countermeasures to chemical, biological, radiological and nuclear threats. As you indicated, I am the Assistant to the Secretary of Defense for Nuclear, Chemical and Biological Defense Programs.

Today, I will address the Department's defense process to identify, prioritize, develop and acquire countermeasures to the threats we face today and future threats. I will also provide an update on some of the accomplishments of the medical research program and the Joint Vaccine Acquisition Program. Finally, I will highlight some of our interagency cooperative efforts and following my comments, I welcome questions the subcommittee might have and I will do the best I can to answer them.

In accordance with congressional authority, I serve as the focal point, overseeing the Department's chemical and biological defense research, development and acquisition programs. The Secretary of Defense recently provided direction to enhance the chemical and biological defense posture. The resulting study generated several options for increased investment based on these new requirements and accompanying risk.

Based on the study findings, senior leaders agreed to increase the investment for WMB countermeasures by $2.1 billion for the fiscal years 2006–2011. The increase included $1.3 billion for Chemical and Biological Defense Program. This investment strategy begins in fiscal year 2006 with $1.5 billion for the President's budget request.

In addition to this study, the Director of Program Analysis and Evaluation identified an additional $100 million in fiscal year 2006 for the Chemical and Biological Defense Program to address biological warfare and medical countermeasure initiatives. These medical countermeasure initiatives will apply transformational approaches which leverage our genomics, proteomics consistent biology data exploitation.

The Chemical and Biological Defense Program has made progress in several areas of medical defense. In 2003, the first successful application of the new animal efficacy rule occurred with Food and Drug Administration approval of pyridostigmine bromide to increase survival exposure to soman nerve agent poisoning.

In March 2005, a contract award was made for development of a chemical agent bioscavenger for a pre or post-exposure treatment of nerve agent exposure. In February of this year, the FDA approved the DOD Vaccinia Immune Globulin used to treat adverse events following smallpox immunization. In early 2005, clinical trials began for both a multivalent botulinium vaccine for stereotypes A and B and a plague vaccine. In July clinical trials will begin for a Venezuelan Equine Encephalitis vaccine.

The DOD Chemical and Biological Defense Program activities are informally coordinated with the Department of Health and Human Services. Stewart Simonson and I meet on a regular basis with the National Institute of Allergy and Infectious Diseases with Dr. Fauci and the Centers for Disease Control and Prevention.

DOD and the DHS are currently working on an interagency agreement regarding cooperation on medical countermeasure development. It is important to note that some of the medical countermeasures currently being developed through NIAID for the national stockpile have their technology bases and programs which initially began in the Department of Defense. Examples of this are the next generation anthrax vaccine and self-culture derived smallpox vaccine.

A critical aspect of interagency coordination is DOD's support for Project BioShield. The first product that DOD may be able to transition to the Department of Health and Human Services under Project BioShield is a plasma-derived, bioscavenger for pre and post-exposure treatment of nerve agent exposure. The DOD has awarded an initial contract for a Phase I clinical trial at which time DHHS would be expected to assume advanced development through FDA licensure under the BioShield authority.

The joint project manager for the Chemical and Biological Medical System is responsible for systems acquisition, production and medical countermeasures against chemical and biological agents, including the Joint Vaccine Acquisition Program. In February of this year, the Under Secretary of Defense for Acquisition Technology and Logistics provided you with a detailed update on the JVAP acquisition program.

The Chemical and Biological Events Program budget provides a balanced investment strategy which includes the procurement of capabilities to protect U.S. forces in the near term, investment in advanced development to protect U.S. forces in the mid term and investment in the science and technology base to protect U.S. forces in the far term and beyond.

As we look to the future, our main concern is a bioengineered threat to our men and women in uniform. Our main task continues to be to provide the best technology to the war fighter in the most expeditious and efficient manner possible. Therefore, my office will continue to focus on providing the technology necessary to counter the threats posed by chemical and biological agents, especially the biological agents.

Thank you for the opportunity to address these issues and I will attempt to answer any questions and concerns the committee might have.

[The prepared statement of Dr. Klein follows:]

REVISED 06/13/05 – WHITE HOUSE

TESTIMONY OF

DR. DALE KLEIN

ASSISTANT TO THE SECRETARY OF DEFENSE

FOR NUCLEAR AND CHEMICAL AND BIOLOGICAL DEFENSE PROGRAMS

BEFORE THE

U.S. HOUSE OF REPRESENTATIVES

COMMITTEE ON GOVERNMENT REFORM

NATIONAL SECURITY, EMERGING THREATS, AND INTERNATIONAL

RELATIONS SUBCOMMITTEE

JUNE 14, 2005

Dr. Dale Klein,
Assistant to the Secretary of Defense
for Nuclear and Chemical and Biological Defense Programs
on
"Elusive Antidotes: Progress Developing Chemical Biological Radiological Nuclear
(CBRN) Countermeasures"

Chairman Shays, Representative Kucinich, and Members of the Committee:

I am honored to appear before your Committee again to address your questions

regarding the Department's efforts to develop and acquire countermeasures to chemical,

biological, radiological, and nuclear (CBRN) threats. I am Dr. Dale Klein, the Assistant

to the Secretary of Defense for Nuclear and Chemical and Biological Defense Programs.

In my testimony today, I will address the Department of Defense's process for

linking our strategic guidance to capabilities, including the process to identify, prioritize,

and develop and acquire countermeasures to the threats that we face today and that we

anticipate facing in the future. I will also provide an update on some of the

accomplishments in the medical research program and the Joint Vaccine Acquisition

Program. Finally, I will highlight some of our interagency cooperative efforts.

Following my comments, I welcome any questions the Committee may have and I

will do my best to answer them.

DoD Chemical and Biological Defense Program — From Strategy to Programs

In accordance with Congressional authority, I serve as focal point overseeing the

Department's chemical and biological defense research, development, and acquisition. In preparation of the Fiscal Year 2006 President's Budget Submission for the Department's Chemical and Biological Defense Program, we used a new process based on the program reorganization that occurred in 2003. This improved process ensures that the Department's efforts in CBRN defense are closely aligned with strategic guidance and are driven by operational requirements, rather than being driven by technological approaches.

The planning process for the budget begins with the *National Security Strategy*, which establishes the position of the United States and outlines the defense strategy. Drawing from the direction and goals in NSS, the Joint Chiefs of Staff prepare and present the *National Military Strategy*. The *National Military Strategy* recommends military objectives and strategy, fiscally constrained force levels, and force options; and provides a risk assessment for programs.

A major aspect of the planning phase is the Joint Capabilities Development process. The Joint Capabilities Development approach to defense planning serves to focus attention on required capabilities while providing guidance to fit programs within the resources available and meet the defense goals. As stated in the guidance, a key Strategic Objective for the Department is to **Secure the United States from Direct Attack**—We will give top priority to dissuading, deterring, and defeating those who seek to harm the United States directly, including those extremist individuals or organizations that may possess and employ weapons of mass destruction.

The current CBRN Defense strategy emphasizes a capabilities-based approach rather than the previous approach, which provided greater emphasis on prioritizing threat agents and targeting budgetary resources based on validated intelligence. Capabilities-based planning focuses more on <u>how</u> adversaries may challenge us than on whom those adversaries might be or where we might face them. It reduces the dependence on intelligence data and recognizes the impossibility of predicting complex events with precision. This strategy drives a top-down, competitive process that enables the Secretary to balance risk across the range of complex threats facing military personnel, to balance risk between current and future challenges, and to balance risk within fiscal constraints.

I appreciate the Congress' support of the FY2005 National Defense Authorization Act. I believe it is worth quoting from the Congressional report language since the rationale coincides with the Department's approach:

The current law [10 USC 2370a] defines biological warfare threats primarily in intelligence terms. This is overly restrictive because intelligence on biological warfare threats is inherently limited due to the ease with which biological warfare programs can be concealed and dangerous pathogens and toxins can be acquired. The situation is further exacerbated by the rapid advancements in bio-technology that are widely available throughout the world. Additionally, the current law categorizes biological warfare agents by the time period in which they may become threats: near-, mid-, and far-term. For the same reasons that make it difficult to define biological warfare agents in terms of available intelligence, it is difficult to project the time periods during which such agents might become threats. In responding to such threats, more flexibility is needed in the medical components of the biological defense research program.

Key capabilities within the Chemical and Biological Defense Program are structured within the operational elements of Sense, Shape, Shield and Sustain.

- *Sense* includes advanced remote sensing, standoff detection and identification systems.

- *Shape* includes battlespace management, including modeling and simulation and the communication and decision systems to make appropriate responses and plans.

- *Shield* includes collective and individual protection and preventive medicines, such as vaccines.

- *Sustain* includes capabilities for decontamination and medical diagnostics and therapeutics.

This approach focuses on optimizing materiel solutions for CBRN defense by building a *portfolio of capabilities* that is robust and agile across the spectrum of requirements, including requirements to support homeland security.

Enhancing Countermeasures

As a supplement to the Joint Capabilities Development process, the Secretary of Defense provided direction to enhance the chemical and biological defense posture. The Joint Requirements Office for CBRN Defense and the Office of the Deputy Assistant to the Secretary of Defense for Chemical and Biological Defense led a comprehensive study that generated several options for increased investment based on the new requirements and accompanying risk. The study used an analytical methodology to define requirements for each Service and for the total requirement for the Joint force.

Based on the study findings, senior leaders agreed to increase the investment for WMD countermeasures by $2.1 billion in Fiscal Years 2006–2011. This increase includes $800 million in military construction funding included in the Defense Health Program for a recapitalization of the facilities at the U.S. Army Medical Research Institute of Infectious Diseases (USAMRIID). The increase also included $1.3 billion for the Chemical and Biological Defense Program, bringing the total chemical and biological defense investment to $9.9 billion over that period. This investment strategy begins with the $1.5 billion FY 06 President's Budget Request. The Chemical and Biological Defense Program increase includes activities to enhance warfighter defense capabilities to include building a new test chamber for non-traditional agents; upgrading test and evaluation facilities; enhancing research and development efforts in areas of agent detection, early warning and battle management, decontamination, collective protection, and medical countermeasures.

The FY06 President's Budget Submission for the DoD Chemical and Biological Defense Program builds on the strategy and the existing capabilities fielded to protect U.S. forces against CBRN threats and includes the results of the study and biological warfare medical countermeasure initiatives. The Chemical and Biological Defense Program budget provides a *balanced investment strategy* that includes the procurement of capabilities to protect U.S. forces in the near-term (FY06), investment in advanced development to protect U.S. forces in the mid-term (FY07–11), and investment in the science and technology base to protect U.S. forces through the far term (FY12–19) and beyond. The two primary areas of increased emphasis in this year's budget are the CB Defense Program's test and evaluation infrastructure and novel biodefense initiatives.

This budget is based on technology needs and directions, restructured acquisition programs, and integrated Test & Evaluation (T&E) capabilities to execute these programs. The programs are time and funding sequenced to be executable in terms of having the technologies demonstrated and transitioned in synchronization with the T&E capabilities. Thus, the milestones of the acquisition programs are based on the availability of not only the financial resources, but the technology and T&E resources needed to execute the programs. The full effect of this integrated, executable program structure will begin to be realized in FY06.

Medical Countermeasures

In addition to the increase mentioned before, the FY06 President's Budget submission included an additional $100 million for the CBDP to address biological warfare medical countermeasure initiatives. Of this funding, approximately 76% is applied to science and technology (S&T) efforts and approximately 24% is applied to advanced development efforts. These medical countermeasure initiatives will apply transformational approaches which leverage genomics, proteomics and systems biology data exploitation. The focus of these biodefense initiatives is on interrupting the disease cycle before and after exposure, as well as countering bioengineered threats.

The Chemical and Biological Defense Program has made progress in several areas of medical defense. I will briefly describe some recent successes. In 2003, the first successful application of the new "animal efficacy rule" occurred with Food and Drug Administration (FDA) approval of pyridostigmine bromide to increase survival after exposure to soman nerve agent poisoning. Evidence from animal models shows that administration of the drug before exposure to soman, together with atropine and pralidoxime given after exposure, increases survival. The FDA agreed that, based on the animal evidence of effectiveness, pyridostigmine bromide is likely to benefit humans exposed to soman. The safety of pyridostigmine bromide has been documented over years of clinical use in the treatment of the neuromuscular disease, *myasthenia gravis*.

In March 2005, a contract award was made for development of a chemical agent bioscavenger for a pre- or post-exposure treatment of nerve agent exposure. This bioscavenger is being developed as a prophylactic regimen to protect the warfighter from incapacitation and death caused by organophosphorus nerve agents.

On the biological side, in early 2005, clinical trails began for a multivalent botulinum vaccine for serotypes A and B, and a plague vaccine; while in July, clinical trials will begin for Venezuelan Equine Encephalitis Vaccine.

Joint Vaccine Acquisition Program

The Joint Project Manager for Chemical Biological Medical Systems is responsible for systems acquisition, production, and deployment of FDA-approved medical countermeasures against chemical and biological agents for the Department of Defense, including the Joint Vaccine Acquisition Program (JVAP).

In February of this year, the Under Secretary of Defense for Acquisition, Technology, and Logistics provided you with a detailed update on the Joint Vaccine Acquisition Program to include vaccines being developed, yearly accomplishments of the program, and funding details. There are no new developments to report at this time.

Near-term (FY06–07) biological medical countermeasure goals include transition to advanced development of bacterial (plague), and viral (Venezuelan Equine Encephalitis (VEE)) vaccines.

Mid-term (FY08–11) opportunities include advanced development of filovirus and ricin toxin vaccines, potential FDA approval of a reduced dosing schedule for the current anthrax vaccine and a Botulinum A/B neurotoxin vaccine.

Long-term (FY12–20) targets include licensure of all near-term and mid-term vaccine candidates in advanced development to include Eastern and Western Equine Encephalitis (EEE and WEE) and combined filovirus vaccines. Furthermore, the program is investigating several alternatives to hypodermic needles for administration of vaccines, which will greatly reduce the medical logistics burden and cost associated with vaccination, and improve user compliance. Another thrust is to identify effective adjuvants to reduce the time and vaccine dose required for development of effective protective immunity. A strategic thrust is to develop innovative multi-agent vaccines that simultaneously target multiple pathogens through a single immunization series. This effort is supported by the investment the program is making in science and technology.

Major technical challenges in the medical pretreatments capability area include defining appropriate *in vitro* and *in vivo* model systems for investigative purposes, determining mechanisms of action of the threat agents, identifying appropriate immunogenic protective antigens for vaccine targets, and stimulating immune responses to small molecules. In addition, other challenges are selecting vector systems for recombinant protein vaccines, evaluating preliminary safety and efficacy data, determining dose and route of administration, and evaluating process-scale up potential. The development of acceptable animal efficacy models is essential to obtain FDA licensure of medical CBD pretreatments, because challenging humans with chemical and biological threat agents to establish vaccine protective efficacy is unethical and prohibited.

Products currently licensed and procured under the JVAP are Anthrax Vaccine Adsorbed (AVA) and Vaccinia Immune Globulin IV, and Dryvax smallpox vaccine. More specifically, JVAP is developing the vaccines below for eventual FDA licensure, listed along with significant program milestones and events. The status of each follows:

- **Plague** vaccine: Phase 1 clinical trial is being conducted at the University of Kentucky, Lexington, KY. The Phase 1 clinical trial started on January 25, 2005.

- **Recombinant Botulinum (rBOT) A/B** vaccine: Phase 1 clinical trial is being conducted at the University of Kentucky, Lexington, KY. The Phase 1 clinical trial started on August 30, 2004.

- **Venezuelan Equine Encephalitis (VEE)** vaccine: A Phase 1 clinical trial will be conducted at Radiant Research, Austin, TX. The Phase 1 clinical trial is scheduled to start in July 2005.

- **Vaccinia Immune Globulin Intravenous (VIG-IV)**: VIG-IV was licensed by the FDA. The FDA issued an approval letter to DVC on February 18, 2005 to market Vaccinia Immune Globulin Intravenous (human) (VIG-IV).

Interagency Program Coordination

The DoD Chemical and Biological Defense Program activities are informally coordinated with the Department of Health and Human Services, including the National Institute of Allergy and Infectious Diseases (NIAID), and the Centers for Disease and Control & Prevention and the Food and Drug Administration. This coordination is evident by the DoD's active participation in the monthly DHHS Risk Management meetings for anthrax, smallpox, and botulinum toxin.

The DynPort Vaccine Company (DVC) is the DoD prime systems contractor for vaccine development. NIAID also funds DVC for some collaborative vaccine efforts. These awards included two grants to support the development of a vaccine candidate for botulinum toxin, a grant to support a Phase II trial of a Venezuelan Equine Encephalitis vaccine, and a contract to fund research on a vaccine candidate for tularemia.

It is important to note that some of the medical countermeasures currently being developed through CDC for the national stockpile have their technology basis in programs which originated in DoD. Examples are the next generation anthrax vaccine and cell culture derived smallpox vaccine. As such, DoD and CDC work cooperatively to leverage medical countermeasure programs of mutual interest including the role played by the DVC for such development. Both DoD and CDC have reviewed their programs to ensure there is no funding redundancy.

DOD and HHS are coordinating efforts to demonstrate the efficacy of antibiotics against plague in animal models.

Management of the development and implementation of national security policies related to CBRN defense activities by multiple agencies of the U.S. Government are coordinated by the joint Homeland Security Council/National Security Council's Policy Coordination Committee for Biodefense. The DoD is represented on this Coordinating Committee.

A critical aspect of interagency coordination is DoD support for Project BioShield. As I testified before the House Government Reform Committee in April 2003, the Department of Defense supported this effort and it has lead to action. The first product that DoD may be able to transition to the Department of Health and Human Services under Project BioShield is the plasma derived bioscavenger. The DoD has awarded an initial contract to the plasma derived bioscavenger in Phase I clinical trials, and upon completion, it may be eligible for procurement by the Department of Health and Human Services under Project BioShield.

Thank you for the opportunity to address these issues. I will try to address any additional concerns or questions the Committee may have.

Mr. SHAYS. Thank you, Dr. Klein.
Dr. Fauci.

STATEMENT OF DR. ANTHONY S. FAUCI

Dr. FAUCI. Thank you for giving me the opportunity to discuss with you this afternoon the NIH biomedical research effort in the development of countermeasures against three major threats, biological, mainly microbes and toxins; radiologic and nuclear countermeasures as well as chemical countermeasures.

We began this endeavor over 3 years ago with the biological and the medical countermeasures including radiologic, nuclear and chemical based on the fundamental basic scientific approach that has been adapted at the NIH for decades in our research in other areas. This includes most recently an expansion of the research capacity, both intellectual capacity of individuals involved as well as physical structure and laboratories. All of these are directed at the development of countermeasures in the form of diagnostics, vaccines and therapeutics.

The greatest success thus far has been in an area in which we have had decades of experience in confronting emerging and re-emerging infectious diseases at our NIH programs. In the end of 2001 and early 2002, following the anthrax attacks, we developed a comprehensive, strategic plan and a research agenda for Category A as well as Category B and C agents. In addition, we have developed and published now for your perusal the progress reports for the Category A agents and most recently, we have included the progress reports for the Category B and C agents.

I would like to spend just a moment or two summarizing some of these accomplishments that have occurred over the past 3 years. First, in the arena of smallpox, you may recall right after the anthrax attack when we examined our stockpile, we had about 15,000–18,000 doses which with dilution brought us up to 90,000. Now, with the techniques that were developed and Dr. Klein just mentioned, we have over 300 million doses of smallpox. In addition, we are working on clinical trials in the next generation, safer, modified vaccinia Ankara as well as antiviral drugs against smallpox.

As was mentioned, the anthrax situation is based on research that is involved in the recombinant protective antigen which has now been contracted for the stockpile through Project BioShield. In addition, we are developing monoclonal and polyclonal antibodies. We have success with Ebola. The Ebola vaccine developed at NIH has proved 100 percent effective in monkeys in protecting them from a challenge. We have just completed a Phase I trial in humans showing it to be safe and immunogenic. Botulism toxin, we are accelerating the development of antibodies, particularly monoclonal antibodies and influenza, which is a Category C agent, we are now well into clinical trials for the H–5 N–1 pandemic flu threat that we now face in Asia. This work is built upon the decades of experience with emerging and a reemerging microbes.

With regard to nuclear countermeasures, this is one that is not as mature in the sense of development of countermeasures from a new standpoint as has the microbes because of the fact this was fundamentally a cold war issue that was developed through the Department of Defense and over the last several years following the dissolution of the cold war threat, we have had to revitalize the program. We are doing that in collaboration with the Department of Defense.

We have a strategic plan for radiologic and nuclear countermeasure development which will be available and was signed off just last night and will be available to you. It includes our intermediate as well as our long range goals. The low hanging fruit is to expand the licensure for material that is already in the strategic national stockpile as well as to develop centers of excellence.

In addition, we are developing protectants as well as response agents and importantly a program to use adult stem cell reconstitution of bone marrow suppression following a radiologic attack. We are using the expertise that was developed in fighting cancer in which one gets exposed to radiation deliberately to kill cancer cells, there is the effect on the bone marrow which we are now using that expertise to try and develop reconstitution.

The same can be said about chemical countermeasures. We have a strategic plan that is not as mature as the radio-biological one. This will likely be available at the end of this calendar year and it is based on the same situation as I mentioned in looking at what we already have in the strategic stockpile and trying to expand the FDA-approved usage of that.

We are doing this in very strong partnership with the U.S. Army Medical Research Institute of Chemical Defense. Again, we have immediate, intermediate and long term goals. The long term goal is to ultimately develop countermeasures that can be used both to detect as well as to counter the effects of tissue damage due to chemical weapons.

Finally, on this last poster, I want to mention the coordination and the collaboration among the various agencies to which the chairman alluded. At the NIH, we coordinate through my institute by a Biodefense Research Coordinating Committee. That is within the NIH institutes as a whole. Much, if not all of the biological microbial is done through the Infectious Disease Institute but when you get into chemical and radiologic, we have a number of the other Institutes at the NIH and we coordinate that through our committee.

The coordination within HHS as you will hear from Assistant Secretary Stewart Simonson takes place in his office at the Office of Public Health Emergency Preparedness and the more global Federal Government coordination among agencies including DHS, DHHS, DOD and others takes place through the Homeland Security Council, particularly through the Weapons of Mass Destruction Medical Countermeasures Subcommittee.

I am finished with the oral statement. I would be happy to answer questions later.

[The prepared statement of Dr. Fauci follows:]

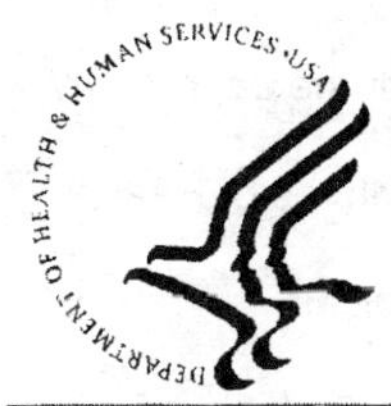

Testimony
Before the Committee on Government Reform
Subcommittee on National Security, Emerging
Threats, and International Relations
United States House of Representatives

The Role of NIH Biomedical Research in Responding to the Threats of Chemical, Biological, Radiological and Nuclear (CBRN) Terrorism

Statement of

Anthony S. Fauci, M.D.

Director
National Institute of Allergy and Infectious Diseases
National Institutes of Health
U.S. Department of Health and Human Services

For Release on Delivery
Expected at 2:00PM
Tuesday, June 14, 2005

Introduction

Mr. Chairman and Members of the Subcommittee, thank you for the opportunity to speak with you today concerning the role of the National Institutes of Health (NIH) in conducting research to further the development of medical countermeasures to protect civilians against attacks using biological, chemical and radiological or nuclear weapons.

I will briefly outline the status of NIH's research and development program in each of these three areas, including a sketch of the strategic planning process that guides the program and a few examples of recent accomplishments. I will then summarize how NIH research in these three areas is coordinated with research conducted by other Federal agencies.

The events of September and October of 2001 clearly exposed the vulnerability of the United States to acts of terrorism that employ unconventional weapons or tactics. In particular, the anthrax attacks made it clear that the potential for terrorist use of deadly pathogens or biological toxins such as those that cause anthrax, smallpox or botulism represents a serious threat. The Administration and Congress immediately responded to this threat by a number of initiatives including significantly increasing funding for research to develop medical countermeasures against a wide variety of biological agents.

Because the National Institute of Allergy and Infectious Diseases (NIAID), a component of the NIH, has for decades played a central role in the conduct of research on emerging and re-emerging infectious diseases, the Institute was chosen to take the lead in Federal research to develop new and improved vaccines, drugs, and diagnostic tools to counter deliberate attacks with biological agents.

We also face other unconventional threats in addition to those from biological agents. These include threats from chemical weapons or toxic industrial compounds; ionizing radiation from the deliberate release of radioactive materials; or, in a worst case scenario, a nuclear explosion of a stolen or improvised nuclear device. NIH has recently been tasked with developing medical countermeasures appropriate for the civilian population for chemical, radiological and nuclear threats, in addition to biological threats. Because NIAID has extensive experience and expertise in developing medical countermeasures against biological agents, it was assigned the role of guiding and coordinating these NIH efforts.

The development of medical countermeasures against non-infectious disease threats presents a different set of scientific challenges that require additional technical expertise and institutional experience. To maintain these distinctions, in my testimony today I will use the terms "biological countermeasures research," "chemical countermeasures research," and "radiological and nuclear countermeasures research," to refer to research for medical countermeasures to infectious agents or toxins, chemical agents, and ionizing radiation, respectively.

NIH Biological Countermeasures Research

The NIH research agenda for defense against threats from infectious agents or biological toxins was developed through a comprehensive strategic planning process initiated in late 2001. In February 2002, NIAID convened a meeting of the *Blue Ribbon Panel on Bioterrorism and Its Implications for Biomedical Research*, whose members were distinguished experts from academic centers, private industry, civilian government agencies, and the military. Three key documents were developed based on this Panel's advice and on extensive discussions with other Federal agencies: the *NIAID Strategic Plan for Biodefense Research, the NIAID Research Agenda for CDC Category A Agents* (for those agents that pose the gravest threat), and the *NIAID Research Agenda for CDC Category B and C Priority Pathogens* (agents whose biological properties make them more difficult to deploy or less likely to cause widespread harm). These documents are available on the NIAID biodefense research program website at http://www2.niaid.nih.gov/biodefense/research/strat_plan.htm.

The *Strategic Plan* provides a blueprint for the conduct of basic research on microbes and host immune defenses, as well as targeted, milestone-driven development of drugs, vaccines, diagnostics and other interventions and resources that would be needed in the event of a bioterror attack. The two biodefense research agendas describe short-term, intermediate, and long-term goals for research on the wide variety of agents that could be used to conduct such an attack. Two recent progress reports describe the significant progress made toward the goals set forth in these research agendas.

The NIH biodefense research agenda encompasses expansion of biodefense infrastructure, basic research, and medical countermeasures development. Overall, the effort to develop new countermeasures rests on a foundation of basic research needed to better understand how pathogens interact with human hosts. For example, one major NIAID basic biodefense research initiative is focused on the human innate immune system, which is comprised of broadly active "first responder" cells and other non-specific mechanisms that are the first line of defense against infection. The development of methods to boost innate immune responses could lead to the development of a relatively small set of fast-acting countermeasures that would be effective against a wide variety of pathogens or toxins that could be used in an attack.

NIH biodefense research is ultimately directed toward the creation of new and effective medical countermeasures, including vaccines, therapeutics, and diagnostics against potential bioterror agents. Substantial progress toward these goals has already been achieved. In the area of therapeutics, for example, NIAID-supported scientists recently discovered that smallpox virus may be halted by aiming a drug not at the virus, but at the cellular machinery the virus needs to spread from cell to cell; this approach might completely circumvent the problem of antiviral drug resistance, and might also be applicable to other viruses. Researchers supported by NIAID also are investigating the use of antibodies that can bind to and block the action of toxins produced by the anthrax bacterium, as well as botulinum toxin.

New and improved strategies for the development of vaccines against potential bioterror agents are being vigorously pursued, with the objective of adding them to the Strategic National Stockpile (SNS) as quickly as possible. For example, NIAID played a major role in the rapid development of the next-generation anthrax vaccine known as recombinant protective antigen, or rPA. Clinical trials to evaluate rPA are currently underway. To date, the immune responses elicited in humans are similar to those elicited in animal studies, which have demonstrated that the rPA vaccine protected animals against aerosol challenge with anthrax spores. Last November, the Department of Health and Human Services (DHHS) awarded a contract for the acquisition of 75 million doses of rPA vaccine to be held in the Strategic National Stockpile (SNS). NIAID's rPA product development initiatives were instrumental in making the SNS initiative possible.

Our preparedness to respond to an attack using smallpox virus has improved enormously since 2001, when only 90,000 doses of smallpox vaccine were readily available for domestic use. Today, because of clinical research on the dose required to produce immunity and an aggressive acquisition program, more than 300 million doses are held in the SNS. Moreover, NIAID-supported researchers also are testing next-generation smallpox vaccines that may prove to be effective for smallpox and safer than the current smallpox vaccines, thus potentially allowing them to be used by populations that have contraindications for currently available smallpox vaccines, including people with weakened immune systems. One of these, modified vaccinia Ankara (MVA), is based on a strain of the vaccinia virus that causes fewer side effects than the traditional Dryvax vaccinia virus strain because it does not replicate effectively in human cells. Human trials of MVA vaccines are under way at NIH and elsewhere. Encouragingly, vaccine manufacturers Bavarian Nordic and Acambis announced this year that Phase I and Phase II trials demonstrated MVA vaccine to be safe and immunogenic in human volunteers, confirming earlier studies by NIAID intramural scientists and their colleagues showing that MVA protects monkeys and mice from smallpox-like viruses.

NIH also has expanded national biodefense research capabilities by investing in several research infrastructure expansion programs. NIAID has established a nationwide network of Regional Centers of Excellence for Biodefense and Emerging Infectious Diseases Research (RCE). These Centers are now conducting fundamental research on infectious diseases that could be used in bioterrorism, developing diagnostics, therapeutics and vaccines needed for biodefense, and providing training for future biodefense researchers. Two new

RCE awards were announced on June 1, 2005, bringing to ten the total number of RCEs nationwide. In addition, NIAID supports the construction of two National Biocontainment Laboratories, built to Biosafety Level 4 standards and therefore capable of safely containing any pathogen, and nine Regional Biocontainment Laboratories (RBLs) with Biosafety Level 3 facilities. NIAID will also support the construction of another four to five RBLs this year. These high-level research laboratories, some of which are already under construction, will provide the facilities needed to carry out the Nation's expanded biodefense research program with the highest degree of safety and security.

NIH-Supported Radiological/Nuclear Countermeasures Research

Threat scenarios that could result in exposure of civilians to ionizing radiation include contamination of food or water with radioactive material, placement of radiation sources in public locations, detonation of a radiological dispersal device (often referred to as an RDD or a "dirty bomb") that scatters radioactive material over a populated area, and attacks on nuclear power plants or high-level nuclear waste storage facilities. The most dangerous scenario would be the detonation of a nuclear explosive device which, in addition to causing enormous destruction from blast and heat, would produce an intense burst of radiation and large quantities of radioactive "fallout."

In 2004, DHHS tasked NIAID with developing a research program to accelerate the development and deployment of new medical countermeasures against ionizing radiation for the civilian population. Through a organized series of structured meetings and other contacts, NIAID worked to build upon prior experience and ongoing research efforts, including those of NCI, as it gathered input from across the Federal government—including the Centers for Disease Control and Prevention (CDC), the Armed Forces Radiobiology Research Institute (AFRRI), and the Department of Energy (DoE)-affiliated National Laboratories—as well as from experts in industry and academia. These activities contributed to the development of an overarching strategic plan and draft research agenda. NIAID next convened a Blue Ribbon Panel in October 2004 to review the draft strategic plan and refine the research agenda for this program. NIAID then assembled the final planning document, entitled *The NIH Strategic Plan and Research Agenda for Medical Countermeasures against Radiological and Nuclear Threats*. This document is in the final stages of production and will be made available shortly.

This *Strategic Research Plan* and *Agenda* is organized into four sections: (1) basic and translational research on the mechanisms of radiation injury, repair, and restoration that can lead to the identification and characterization of new therapeutics; (2) bioassays and tools for biodosimetry, which will aid in diagnosis; (3) immediate product development of promising therapies; and (4) infrastructure to support the necessary research. The document is intended to unify and strengthen the research community focused on these areas, promote increased collaboration, and facilitate transition from research to product development. NIH will work closely with DHHS to prioritize the research and development activities in this ambitious agenda within the resources available and as one component of the larger National medical countermeasures research agenda.

Even before the *Plan* and *Agenda* were complete, NIH recognized the need to collaborate and work in partnership with other Federal agencies involved with radiological research. For example, through an Interagency Agreement signed in 2003, NIAID assisted AFRRI in the restoration of a Cobalt-60 source of gamma irradiation critical for ongoing animal studies to evaluate the effectiveness of anti-radiation drugs. NIAID continues to work closely with AFRRI on collaborative projects involving biodosimetry and promising therapeutics.

NIAID also works closely with our sister Institute at NIH, the National Cancer Institute (NCI), on medical issues involving radiation. Since NCI is involved with therapeutic applications of radiation in the treatment of cancer and has similar concerns about the hazardous effects of ionizing radiation on normal cells and tissues, a partnership effort has evolved that brings together the scientific strengths of NIAID in immunology with those of NCI in therapeutic radiation oncology.

Funding for NIH radiation countermeasures research in fiscal year (FY) 2005 is $47 million; these funds are provided through an appropriation to the Public Health and Social Services Emergency Fund in the Office of the Secretary and are not part of the annual NIH budget. A proposal for specific project commitments for FY 2005 funds has recently been discussed within the Department. The *Strategic Plan* will be reviewed periodically and modified as necessary, subject to progress toward specific milestones.

NIH-Supported Chemical Countermeasures Research

A wide variety of chemicals, with a broad range of toxicities and harmful effects, could be employed in an attack on the civilian population. Threat scenarios include the release of illegally obtained or manufactured chemical warfare agents, the release of purchased or stolen industrial chemicals, and attacks on chemical manufacturing plants, storage sites, or transport vehicles. Some of the many challenges that require medical countermeasures include:

- neurotoxic chemicals, such as organophosphates, that have a direct and deadly effect on the central nervous system;
- vesicating agents, such as mustard gas, that cause skin blisters, blindness, and airway injury;
- metabolic poisons, such as cyanide, that can be inhaled or ingested and lead to death within a matter of minutes or days; and
- lung-damaging liquids and gases, such as chlorine and phosgene, two commonly used industrial chemicals.

The FY 2006 President's Budget requests $50 million for this research. DHHS recently tasked NIAID with drafting a strategic plan and research agenda to guide development of medical countermeasures against chemical threats, in an effort similar in scope and purpose to that for radiological/nuclear countermeasures. Building on an NIAID expert panel convened in 2003 to review the current state of medical chemical defense research, NIAID recently held two focused expert workshops on countermeasure development, one to examine countermeasures for cyanide poisoning and another to assess anticonvulsant drugs that could be used in nerve agent poisoning to prevent and treat seizures. A third workshop on therapies for pulmonary edema is scheduled for August of this year. Ideas developed at these meetings will be incorporated into a Strategic Plan and Research Agenda, which is expected to be complete by the end of this calendar year.

Throughout this process, NIAID has collaborated closely with other Federal agencies. The United States Army Medical Research Institute for Chemical Defense (USAMRICD), headquartered at the Aberdeen Proving Ground in Maryland, is the primary Department of Defense (DoD) research organization for chemical countermeasures and one of our most important institutional partners in this effort. USAMRICD is part of the U.S. Army Medical Research and Materiel Command headquartered at Fort Detrick, Maryland. It is our intent to continue to work closely with the Army on medical products that could benefit both the civilian and military communities. NIAID also is partnering with several NIH laboratories and exploring collaboration with other NIH Institutes, such as the National Institute of Neurological Disorders and Stroke (NINDS).

Coordination of NIH-Supported Medical Countermeasures Research

Although NIH is a leading agency in government-sponsored research to develop

medical countermeasures against biological, chemical, or radiological terrorist

threats, it is by no means the only agency involved; the CDC, the Food and Drug

Administration (FDA), the DoD, the Department of Homeland Security (DHS), the

Department of Agriculture (USDA), the DoE, and other governmental

organizations also play important roles. Coordination among the various

agencies involved is, therefore, extremely important. In broad terms, NIH-

supported medical countermeasures research activities in all three areas are

coordinated using similar mechanisms, at three distinct levels: within NIH, within

DHHS, and across the government as a whole.

Within NIH. NIAID is responsible for the majority of NIH-sponsored medical

countermeasures research for infectious agents and toxins, although other NIH

Institutes and Centers make significant contributions. Because the immune

system is highly susceptible to damage from radiation, NIAID also is directly

involved in both the planning and conduct of radiological/nuclear

countermeasures research in collaboration with NCI. NIAID's direct role in the

development of chemical countermeasures is more limited, and consists mainly

of planning and coordination of activities. This may change as the civilian

chemical and toxin threats are further defined. The focal point for trans-NIH

coordination and planning of all medical countermeasure research activities in all these areas is the NIH Biodefense Research Coordinating Committee. I am Chairman of this committee, which meets at least quarterly. It is administered by the NIAID Office of Biodefense Research, which also serves as liaison office for NIH contacts with other Federal agencies such as DoD and DHS regarding biodefense research and response.

Within DHHS. At the level of DHHS, coordination of medical countermeasures research between the CDC, NIH, FDA, and other agencies within DHHS is the responsibility of the DHHS Office of the Assistant Secretary for Public Health Emergency Preparedness (ASPHEP). The ASPHEP Office of Research and Development Coordination holds periodic meetings with all governmental stakeholders in the development of medical countermeasures.

Across Federal Agencies. At the highest level, coordination of medical countermeasures research is carried out by the White House, and in particular, the Homeland Security Council and the National Security Council. The focal point for USG interagency efforts to prioritize and coordinate medical countermeasures acquisition programs under Project BioShield s the Weapons of Mass Destruction Medical Countermeasures (WMDMC) Subcommittee ("WMDMC Subcommittee"). Assistant Secretary Simonson of HHS, along with representatives from the Department of Homeland Security (DHS) and the Department of Defense (DoD), co-chairs the WMDMC Subcommittee and stakeholders from throughout the USG are represented on it. Since it is the primary federal agency responsible for the development and acquisition of priority medical countermeasures, HHS has a major leadership role in the WMDMC Subcommittee.

Although these three levels describe the basic structure through which the Nation's biodefense research programs are formally coordinated, NIH collaborates daily with the other Federal agencies and is party to a large number of interagency programs, informal contacts, and communication mechanisms that significantly contribute to the efficiency and effectiveness with which medical countermeasures research is carried out across the U.S. government. For example, members of my staff meet regularly with the research community at Fort Detrick and the United States Army Medical Research and Materiel Command, and with the staff of AFRRI. Through such meetings, synergy in research and mutual support leading to the development of new drugs, vaccines, and diagnostic tests for the nation are achieved. My staff also holds meetings periodically with the Defense Threat Reduction Agency and the Defense Advanced Research Projects Agency, two important entities within the research infrastructure in the DoD.

In order to monitor and understand new threats that may arise, we work closely with DHS and intelligence agencies, which provide threat assessments concerning issues germane to our research. Because new infectious disease challenges emerge naturally on a regular basis, NIH has considerable experience in rapidly mobilizing research resources to confront new infectious disease threats. This experience serves us well when called upon to adjust our research priorities in response to new information.

In closing, although we are concerned and take very seriously the threats of biological, chemical, and nuclear/radiological terrorism, we are confident that our current and planned efforts will lead to new and improved medical countermeasures against these threats. I am also pleased with the degree of coordination and cooperation between NIH and other Federal agencies involved in carrying out these various research programs. Having said that, we will continue to try to improve these interactions.

I appreciate this opportunity to testify before you today, and I would be pleased to answer any questions that you may have.

The Role of NIH Biomedical Research in Responding to the Threats of CBRN Terrorism

Anthony S. Fauci, M.D.
Director
National Institute of Allergy and Infectious Diseases
National Institutes of Health
Department of Health and Human Services

June 14, 2005

House Committee on Government Reform
Subcommittee on National Security, Emerging Threats
and International Relations

NIH Medical Countermeasures Research

- Biodefense Countermeasures

- Radiological and Nuclear Countermeasures

- Chemical Countermeasures

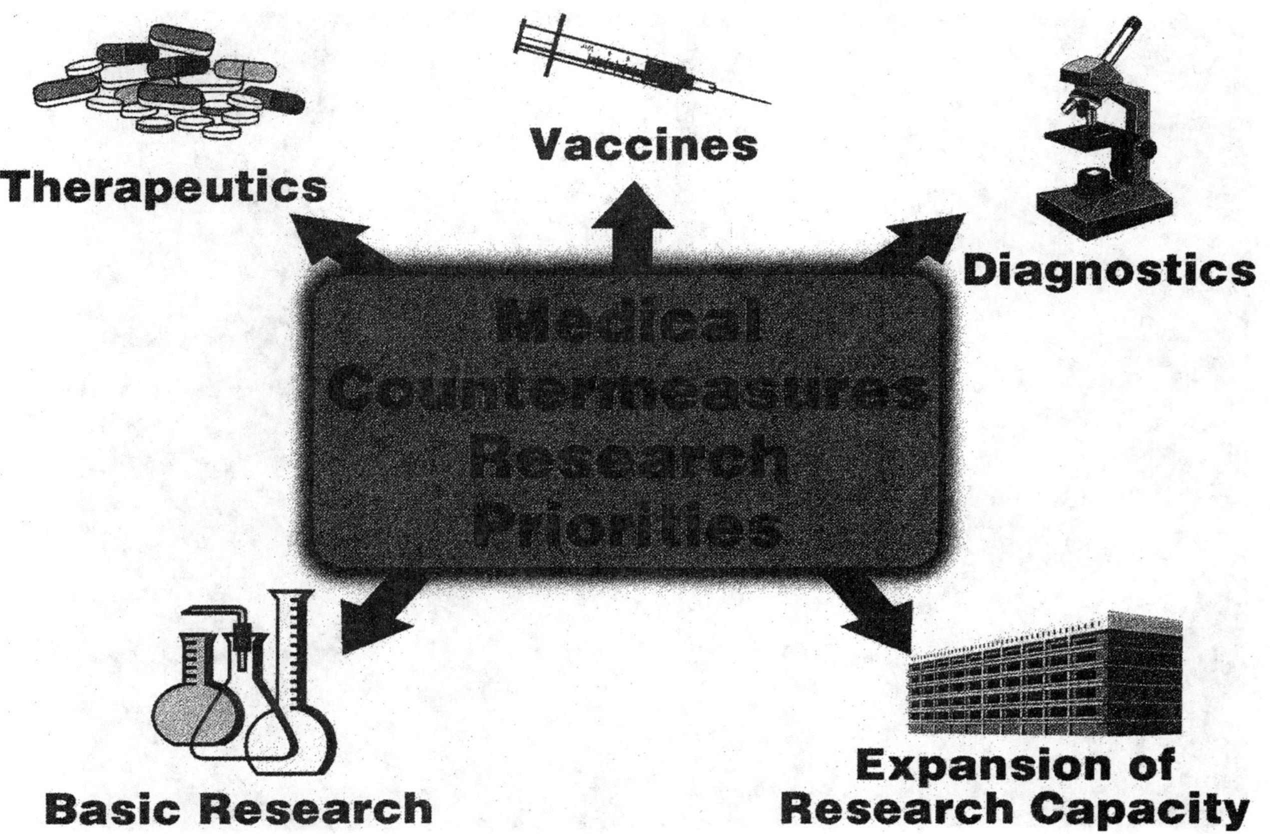

Medical Countermeasures Research Priorities
Therapeutics
Vaccines
Diagnostics
Basic Research
Expansion of Research Capacity

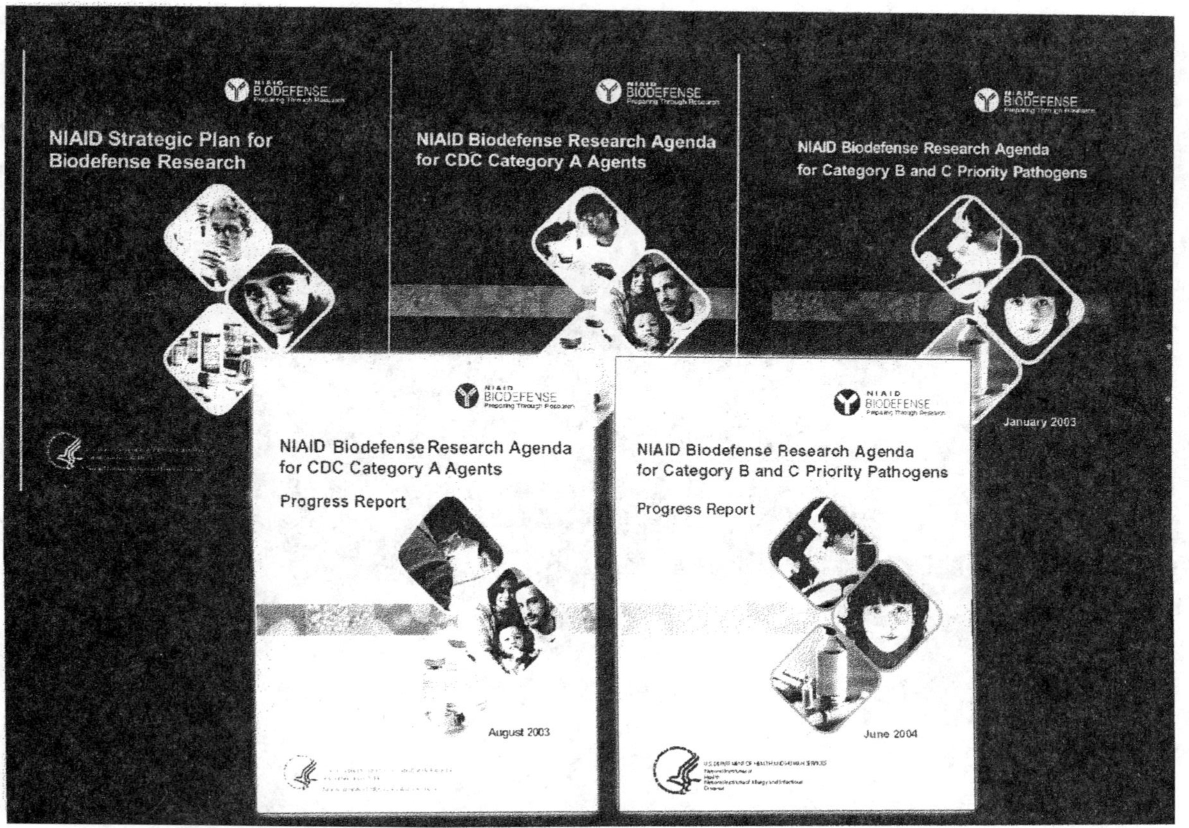
NIAID
BIODEFENSE
Preparing Through Research
NIAID Strategic Plan for
Biodefense Research
NIAID
BIODEFENSE
Preparing Through Research
NIAID Biodefense Research Agenda
for CDC Category A Agents
NIAID
BIODEFENSE
Preparing Through Research
NIAID Biodefense Research Agenda
for Category B and C Priority Pathogens
January 2003
NIAID
BIODEFENSE
Preparing Through Research
NIAID Biodefense Research Agenda
for CDC Category A Agents
Progress Report
August 2003
NIAID
BIODEFENSE
Preparing Through Research
NIAID Biodefense Research Agenda
for Category B and C Priority Pathogens
Progress Report
June 2004
U.S. DEPARTMENT OF HEALTH AND HUMAN SERVICES
National Institutes of Health
National Institute of Allergy and Infectious Diseases

Biodefense Countermeasures: Key Achievements

Smallpox

- More than 300 million doses of smallpox vaccine now available
- "Next-generation" vaccine (MVA) in advanced testing
- Antiviral drug development, e.g. oral cidofovir

Anthrax

- New vaccine (rPA) tested and procured under Project Bioshield
- Development of novel antitoxins, e.g. monoclonal/polyclonal antibodies

Biodefense Countermeasures: Key Achievements (continued)

Ebola

- Vaccine in human trials at NIAID Vaccine Research Center

Botulinum Toxin

- Development of vaccine and monoclonal/polyclonal antibodies

Influenza

- Development of vaccines against potential pandemic strains

Radiological/Nuclear Countermeasures: Research Goals

Immediate

- Facilitate the licensure of drugs in the Strategic National Stockpile by developing animal models and assays

- Develop Centers of Excellence in Radiobiology Research

Intermediate/Long-Term

- Develop broadly acting safe and effective radioprotectant and therapeutic drugs

- Develop biodosimetric tools and bioassays to evaluate radiation injury

- Address critical gaps in understanding mechanisms leading to injury induced by ionizing radiation

- Support stem cell research effort toward reconstitution of immune system following radiation-induced injury

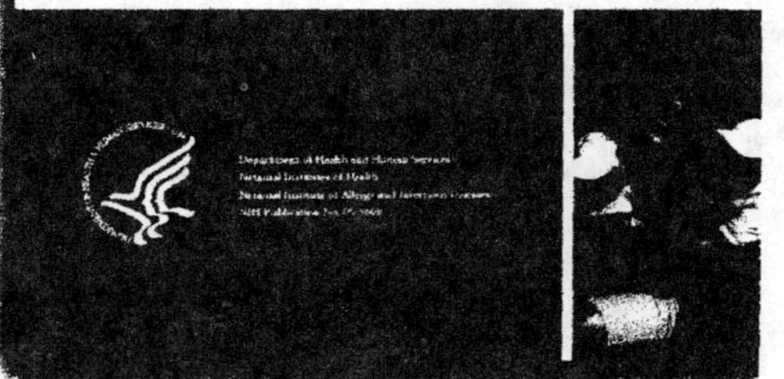

Chemical Countermeasures: Research Goals

Immediate

- Expand indications of FDA-approved drugs for use in treatment of chemical injury
- Develop Centers of Excellence in Medical Chemical Defense Research
- Partner with U.S. Army Medical Research Institute of Chemical Defense (USAMRICD) to expand product development efforts

Intermediate/Long-Term

- Develop broadly acting interventions to prevent and treat chemical injury and to promote recovery
- Develop rapid assessment tools to determine extent of chemical injury and prognosis

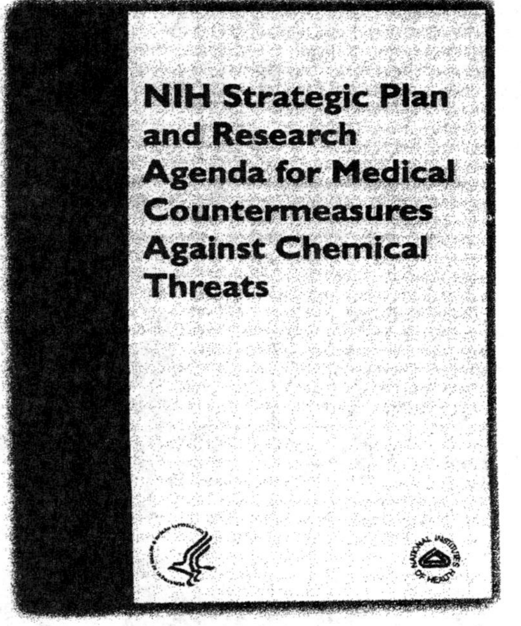

Coordination of Medical Countermeasures Activities

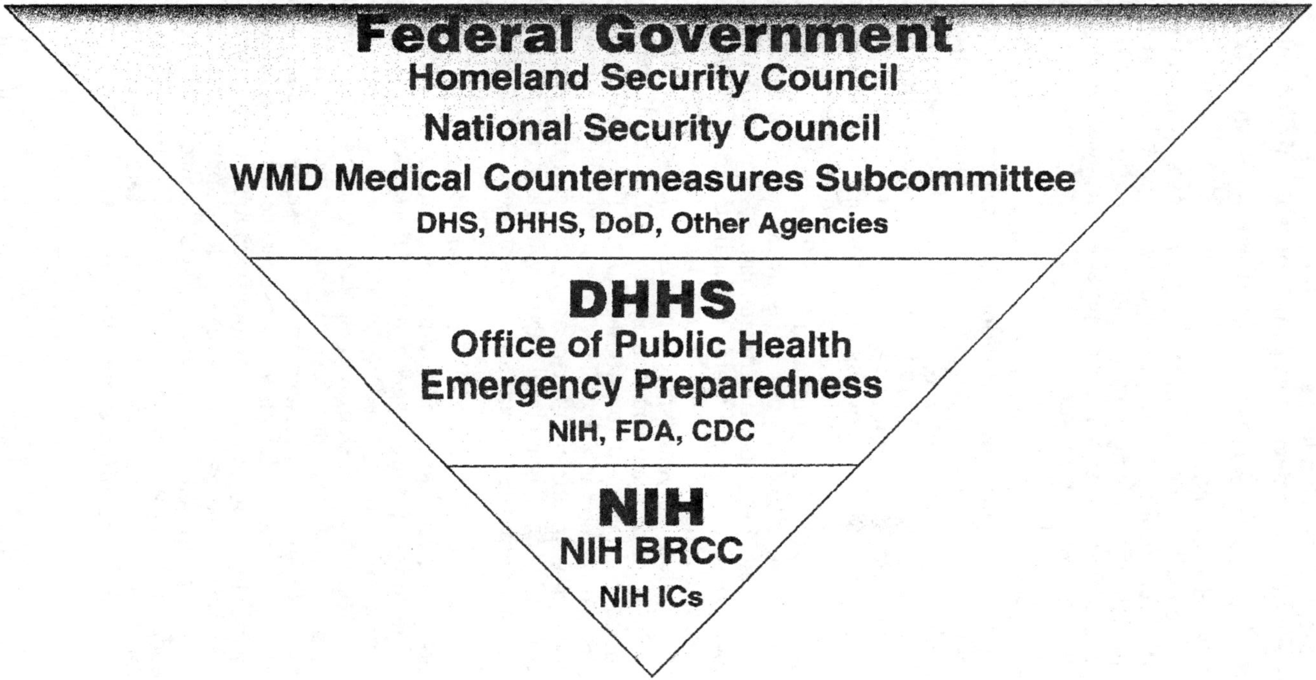

Mr. SHAYS. Thank you.

We have four doctors and an honorable. Mr. Secretary.

STATEMENT OF STEWART SIMONSON

Mr. SIMONSON. Thank you.

Good afternoon. I am Stewart Simonson, Assistant Secretary at HHS for Public Health Emergency Preparedness. I appreciate the opportunity to share with you information on the Department's progress on research development and acquisition programs for medical countermeasures and specifically implementation of the Project BioShield Act of 2004.

HHS shares the subcommittee's desire for an effective and efficient interagency process to identify, prioritize and acquire medical countermeasures to address chemical, biological, radiological and nuclear threat agents. We also share the subcommittee's concern that this process needs to be linked to validated threats.

The events of September and October 2001 made it very clear that terrorism is a serious threat to our Nation and to the world. The Bush administration and Congress responded forcefully to this threat by strengthening our medical and public health capacities to protect our citizens from these attacks. To encourage the development of new medical countermeasures against threat agents and to speed their delivery, President Bush in his 2003 State of the Union Address proposed, and Congress enacted, Project BioShield. The $5.6 billion, 10 year, special reserve fund was created to assure developers of medical countermeasures that funds would be available for the Government to purchase critical products.

Since enactment, my office has moved aggressively to fill immediate gaps in our countermeasures. A genuine sense of urgency informs all of our homeland security work at HHS but it is important to note that the successful development and manufacture of safe and effective countermeasures requires an investment of both money and time. No matter how hard we work or how much money we spend, some steps in the process cannot be rushed.

There is a complex spectrum of efforts needed along the research and development pipeline to produce a usable medical product countermeasure. Defining specifications for a needed countermeasure often reveals few, if any, candidates in the pipeline. To date, we have been fortunate that some of our highest priority needs for medical countermeasures could be addressed using the available, advanced development products in the pipeline.

However, research and early development efforts, even when robustly funded, often take years before a concept is mature enough for advanced development. It is only when a product has reached the advanced development stage that Project BioShield provides a meaningful incentive for manufacturers the product the rest of the way.

In determining the requirements for and elaborating options on medical countermeasure acquisitions, the focal point for U.S. Government interagency efforts is the Weapons of Mass Destruction Countermeasures Subcommittee. HHS, along with representatives from the Department of Homeland Security and the Department of Defense, chair the WMD Subcommittee and stakeholders from throughout the Government are represented on its working groups.

In setting priorities for medical countermeasure acquisitions under BioShield, the WMD Subcommittee considers a number of factors. The credibility and immediacy of the threat are driving factors and our informed by material threat assessments conducted by DHS. We also consider the current and projected availability of appropriate medical countermeasures as well as the target population for which the countermeasure would be used. In addition, logistical issues are considered such as the feasibility of deployment in public health emergencies, shelf life, storage and maintenance requirements.

Project BioShield also requires a number of findings by the Secretaries of Homeland Security and HHS prior to an acquisition commencing. These findings include three determinations: first, that there is a material threat against the U.S. population sufficient to affect national security; second, that the medical countermeasures are necessary to protect the public health from the material threat; and third, that acquiring a specific quantity of a particular countermeasure, using the special reserve fund, is appropriate. These determinations are followed by a joint recommendation to the White House by the two Secretaries. If approved, Congress is notified and HHS executes the acquisition program.

The process that I have outlined has been successfully implemented through contract award three times since the enactment of Project BioShield less than a year ago. HHS has completed contract awards for acquisitions of next generation recombinant protective antigen anthrax vaccine, the current generation licensed anthrax vaccine, and pediatric formulation of potassium iodide. Additionally, the acquisition process is in the final execution phases for several other needed medical countermeasures including anthrax therapeutics, botulinum antitoxin and next generation smallpox vaccine.

This robust interagency process mines the expertise in the scientific and intelligence communities to define requirements for medical countermeasures and enables policymakers to identify and evaluate acquisition options to address immediate and future needs.

In closing, let me say that HHS has a clear mandate from President Bush and Congress to lead the charge in medical countermeasure development. We have already made important strides to address the public health needs of the Nation but more needs to be done. I look forward to working with you and the subcommittee to address the challenges of CBRM preparedness and its importance to public health.

I look forward to answering your questions.

[The prepared statement of Mr. Simonson follows:]

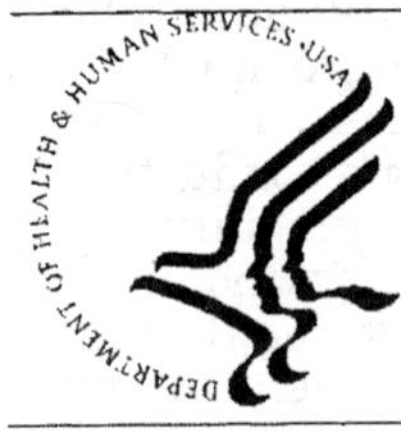

Testimony
Before the Committee on Government Reform
Subcommittee on National Security, Emerging
Threats, and International Relations
United States House of Representatives

The Role of HHS in the Development and Acquisition of Medical Countermeasures for Chemical, Biological, Radiological and Nuclear (CBRN) Threats

Statement of
Stewart Simonson
Assistant Secretary
Office of Public Health Emergency Preparedness
U.S. Department of Health and Human Services

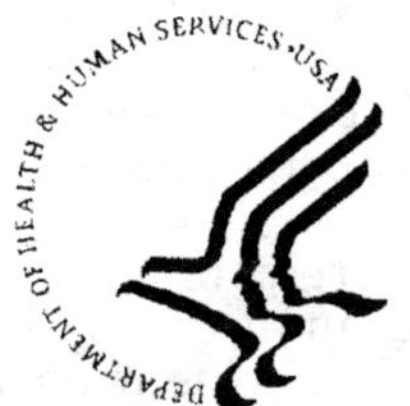

For Release on Delivery
Expected at 2:00 p.m.
Tuesday, June 14, 2005

Good afternoon, Mr. Chairman, Mr. Kucinich and Subcommittee members. I am

Stewart Simonson, Assistant Secretary for Public Health Emergency

Preparedness, Department of Health and Human Services (HHS). I appreciate

the opportunity to share with you information on the Department's progress in

research, development and acquisition programs for medical countermeasures,

particularly with regard to the implementation of the Project BioShield Act of 2004

("Project BioShield"). These programs are vital components of our strategy to

protect the Nation from threats posed from chemical, biological, radiological and

nuclear (CBRN) threats. Defending against such threats is a top priority for the

Bush Administration and having an appropriate armamentarium of medical

countermeasures is a critical element of the response and recovery component

of the President's "21st Century Strategy for Biodefense." The acquisition and

ready availability of medical countermeasures, such as antibiotics, antivirals,

monoclonal and polyclonal antibodies against infectious threats, therapies for

chemical and radiation-induced illnesses, and vaccines to protect against

exposure from biological agents are essential to our Nation's preparedness and

response capabilities.

Protecting Americans

The events of September and October 2001 made it very clear that terrorism-

indeed bioterrorism- is a serious threat to our Nation and the world. The Bush

Administration and Congress responded forcefully to this threat by providing

funding to strengthen our medical and public health capacities to protect our citizens from future attacks. Specifically, substantial increases in funding for research, development and acquisition of medical countermeasures against biological threats were directed to the National Institutes of Health (NIH) and the Centers for Disease Control and Prevention's Strategic National Stockpile (SNS or "the Stockpile"). To further encourage the development of new medical countermeasures against chemical, biological, radiological and nuclear agents and to speed their delivery and use should there be an attack, President Bush, in his 2003 State of the Union address proposed and Congress subsequently enacted Project BioShield. The Special Reserve Fund, appropriated with $5.6 billion was created to assure developers of medical countermeasures that funds would be available to purchase these critical products for use to protect our citizens.

HHS Research Efforts to Respond to CBRN Threats

Dr. Anthony Fauci, the Director of the National Institute of Allergy and Infectious Diseases (NIAID), a component of the NIH, will be testifying here today regarding the role of his institute in research and development of needed medical countermeasures for CBRN threats. NIAID is leading the Federal research enterprise in this area and Dr. Fauci will detail the Institute's efforts. I will focus my testimony on the efforts at HHS to lead the acquisition of medical countermeasures for the SNS.

The Strategic National Stockpile Today

The wake-up call that we received in the fall of 2001 highlighted the gaps in our medical countermeasure armamentarium and we immediately sought to address them. Although much remains to be done, we have made significant progress in building our Strategic National Stockpile from that time to what we have on-hand today. For example, our smallpox vaccine stockpile has grown from 90,000 ready-to-use doses in 2001 to enough vaccine to protect every man, woman, and child in America. Major strides have been made in building our medical countermeasure reserve against anthrax, plague, and tularemia. We are now able to protect and treat millions of Americans in the event of an attack with one of these agents. We have taken the botulinum antitoxin program started by the Department of Defense in the early 1990s to completion and we are now building our botulinum antitoxin stockpile further. We have also built our stockpile of countermeasures to address the effects of radiation exposure with products such as Prussian Blue and diethylenetriaminepentaacetate (DTPA). These countermeasures act to block uptake or remove radioactive elements such as cesium, thallium, or americium from the body after they are ingested or inhaled. Potassium iodide, a drug that can protect the thyroid from the harmful effects of radioactive iodine, is also in the Stockpile.

The Strategic Approach to Addressing Medical Countermeasure Gaps

The initial focus of our efforts to protect the Nation was aimed largely at those threats that could do the greatest harm to the greatest number of our citizens. Among biological threat agents, smallpox and anthrax are widely recognized as having the greatest potential to cause catastrophic harm. A sense of urgency

has pervaded our efforts and we have defined new ways of doing business. Our

new national security environment demands accelerated product development

timelines and new paradigms of interactions between industry and government

with increased risk-sharing and enhanced intra-governmental collaboration.

The focal point for USG interagency efforts to prioritize and coordinate medical

countermeasures acquisition programs is the Weapons of Mass Destruction

Medical Countermeasures (WMDMC) Subcommittee ("WMDMC Subcommittee").

HHS, along with representatives from the Department of Homeland Security

(DHS) and the Department of Defense (DoD), co-chairs the WMDMC

Subcommittee and stakeholders from throughout the USG are represented on it.

Because HHS is the primary federal agency responsible for the development and

acquisition of priority medical countermeasures, we have a major leadership role

in the WMDMC Subcommittee.

The cornerstone of any sound acquisition program is the determination and

prioritization of requirements and this is a primary activity of the WMDMC

Subcommittee. In setting priorities for medical countermeasure acquisition under

Project BioShield, the WMDMC Subcommittee considers a number of factors.

The credibility and immediacy of the specific threats are driving factors and are

informed by Material Threat Assessments (MTAs) conducted by the DHS. Dr.

John Vitko, here today representing DHS, will provide insight into these efforts.

Other factors include an evaluation of the availability of appropriate countermeasures, both current and projected, and the target population for which the medical countermeasure would be used. In addition, logistical issues are considered such as the feasibility of deployment in a public health emergency, shelf life, and the storage and maintenance requirements. Project BioShield also requires a number of findings by the Secretaries of Homeland Security and HHS prior to an acquisition commencing. These findings include:

- Determination of material threat against the US population sufficient to affect national security. This determination is made by the Secretary of Homeland Security.

- Determination that countermeasures are necessary to protect public health. This determination is made by the Secretary of HHS.

- Determination of the appropriateness of funding acquisition of the countermeasure with the Special Reserve Fund (SRF). This determination is made by the Secretary of HHS.

Once these determinations are made, a joint recommendation for the acquisition is presented to the White House by the two Secretaries. If approved, Congress is notified and HHS executes the acquisition program.

The process that I have outlined for you has been successfully implemented three times since the enactment of Project BioShield less than one year ago. HHS has completed contract awards for acquisitions of the next-generation recombinant protective antigen (rPA) anthrax vaccine, the current-generation licensed anthrax vaccine (Anthrax Vaccine Adsorbed, AVA), and the pediatric formulation of potassium iodide. Additionally, the acquisition process is in the final execution phases for several other needed medical countermeasures including anthrax therapeutics, botulinum antitoxin, and a next-generation smallpox vaccine.

This robust interagency process mines the expertise of subject matter experts in the scientific and intelligence communities to define requirements for medical countermeasures and enable policy makers to identify and evaluate acquisition options to address immediate and future needs.

Application of the Strategic Approach: Anthrax.

The efficiency and effectiveness of the steps used to identify, prioritize, and acquire needed medical countermeasures is best exemplified by our efforts to protect the Nation in the event of an anthrax attack. It will also illustrate intra-agency and interagency processes.

Although anthrax is not transmissible from person-to-person, an attack involving the aerosol dissemination of anthrax spores, particularly in an urban setting, is considered by public health experts to have the potential to cause catastrophic damage. The potential for large-scale population exposure following aerosol release of anthrax spores, the threat demonstrated by the anthrax letters, and our knowledge that anthrax had been weaponized by state-actors, highlighted the nature of the threat. The Secretary of Homeland Security determined that anthrax posed a material threat to the Nation. Because untreated inhalation anthrax is usually fatal, the Secretary of HHS identified anthrax as a significant threat to public health.

The approach to protect citizens against this threat demanded immediate, intermediate and long-term strategies and requirements. First, the existing stockpile of antibiotics in the Strategic National Stockpile was increased. Second, there is a need for a licensed vaccine to be used not only for pre-exposure protection for laboratory and other workers at known risk for anthrax, but for use along with antibiotics after an exposure which could decrease the currently recommended 60-day course of antibiotic therapy. Anthrax spores are stable in the environment and would have a profound impact if released in an urban population. Therefore, availability of a vaccine may be a critical requirement for repopulation and restoration of the functionality of any exposed area.

Due to limitations inherent in the currently available anthrax vaccine, there is consensus in the scientific community about the need to develop and acquire a next-generation anthrax vaccine using 21st century technologies An assessment of developing technologies was undertaken by HHS experts in the fall of 2001 and the decision was made that there was a sufficient scientific foundation, including a detailed understanding of the pathogenesis of anthrax and how anthrax vaccines provide protective immunity, to support the aggressive development of a next generation vaccine consisting of recombinant protective antigen (rPA). The research undertaken to develop this vaccine, spanning more than a decade, was conducted in large part by the United States Army Medical Research Institute of Infectious Diseases at Fort Detrick, Maryland.

HHS defined a three-stage development and acquisition strategy with open competition for awards at each stage. The early and advanced development programs were supported by the NIAID with contract awards in September 2002 and 2003, respectively. These were milestone-driven contracts with well-defined deliverables including the manufacture of clinical-grade vaccine, the conduct of Phase I and Phase II clinical trials, and consistency lot manufacturing of vaccine. Large-scale manufacturing capacity would be required to support the civilian requirement for this medical countermeasure, which was defined by the WMD Subcommittee to be the initial protection of up to 25 million persons. Senior officials from several Departments of the USG evaluated acquisition options to achieve this requirement and, in the fall of 2003, approved the decision to pursue this acquisition of rPA anthrax vaccine.

An evaluation of the NIAID rPA anthrax vaccine development program indicated that it was robust enough to suggest that the rPA vaccine could become a licensed product within 8 years. In March 2004, the acquisition program for this vaccine, under the direction of my office, was launched using the Special

Reserve Fund created in the FY 2004 DHS appropriations bill. Utilizing a robust technical and business evaluation process, we reviewed multiple proposals and negotiated a contract for the acquisition of 75 million doses of the vaccine (anticipating a three-dose regimen). Using a milestone and deliverables approach similar to the ACAM2000 smallpox vaccine development and acquisition program, and the rPA anthrax vaccine development contracts at NIAID, the rPA vaccine BioShield acquisition contract lays out an ambitious program for the production of this vaccine. In accordance with Project BioShield, a critical aspect of this acquisition contract is the fact that no payment for product is made until a usable product is delivered to the SNS. While awaiting delivery of the rPA anthrax vaccine to the SNS, my office awarded a contract last month for 5 million doses of the currently licensed AVA vaccine to support immediate requirements. Delivery of this product to the Stockpile began soon after contract award and over one million doses of the licensed anthrax vaccine are now in the SNS.

Application of the Strategic Approach: Other Medical Countermeasures
In an effort to fill other medical countermeasure gaps, we have made progress in contracting for products that are or will soon be delivered to the SNS.
Potassium Iodide.
In March 2005 a contract was awarded under Project BioShield for a pediatric liquid formulation of potassium iodide, a drug that helps limit risk of damage to the thyroid, from radioactive iodine. This formulation is aimed at young children

who have difficulty taking pills and are at the highest risk of harmful effects from exposure to radioactive iodine. This acquisition will provide needed protection for at least 1.7 million children. Product delivery began last month and should be completed by the end of the fiscal year.

Ongoing Project BioShield activities.

In addition to the acquisition contracts that have been awarded since enactment of Project BioShield, there are several other important BioShield procurement-related activities underway. We are engaged in contract negotiations for anthrax therapies, and we are continuing to move forward on the acquisition of an antitoxin treatment for botulism. Furthermore, HHS has moved forward with the initial stages of an acquisition program for a next generation smallpox vaccine to meet a requirement for this product that addresses the millions of U.S. citizens who have contraindications for existing smallpox vaccines. A draft RFP was released last month; the final RFP will be released following review of industry comments. We also anticipate releasing a draft RFP for industry comment next month to address requirements for therapeutics for acute radiation syndrome.

Finally, in anticipation of yet to be determined requirements, we actively monitor the state of the medical countermeasure pipeline-- both within and outside the government--- by evaluating USG research and development portfolios and engaging industry through the publication of Requests for Information (RFIs). For example, we have recently released three RFIs to assess the timeline to maturity of medical countermeasures to treat nerve agent exposure, acute radiation syndrome, and additional products that might be available to treat anthrax. These requests are a key tool for HHS to dialogue with industry partners and to inform the development of sound USG acquisition strategies.

Priority Setting Beyond Smallpox and Anthrax

The approach taken to rapidly expand our Nation's response capacity to meet the medical and public health impact of either a smallpox or anthrax attack demonstrate our national resolve to address these threats. However, in many ways, anthrax and smallpox represent the "low hanging fruit" for medical countermeasure research, development and acquisition and was largely made possible by a substantial research base developed by USAMRIID and NIH. There was consensus that these were our highest priorities and we had countermeasures available or relatively far along in the development pipeline to permit acquisition. Given an almost endless list of potential threats with finite resources to address them, prioritization is essential to focus our efforts. We rely heavily upon our interagency partner, the Department of Homeland Security, to provide us with a prioritized list of threats along with material threat assessments that will include reasonable estimates of population exposure. This information is critical for future strategic decision making regarding how best to focus our National efforts in countermeasure development and acquisition, including whether in the short-term, the so-called "one-bug, one-drug" approach should continue while simultaneously investing in more broad-spectrum prevention and treatment approaches for the longer term.

Novel and Emerging Threats

The initial efforts for medical countermeasure development and acquisition have been rightfully focused on those threat agents known to have the potential to inflict catastrophic harm on our Nation. In addition, HHS and NIH are investing in efforts to address threat agents that we might face in the future, including engineered threats.

As is also the case for the known threat agents, we are dependent upon our colleagues at DHS to identify and prioritize these threats. One of the most recognized potential engineered threats is antibiotic-resistant anthrax, and the HHS, NIH and the U.S. Food and Drug Administration (FDA) accomplishments to date in facilitating the development and acquisition of anthrax vaccines and therapeutic antitoxins have made an important impact on reducing our vulnerabilities in this area. In addition, NIH has made a robust investment in the development of novel antimicrobial agents and in addressing all aspects of antibiotic resistance. For example, investments have been made in the development of antibacterial agents that could potentially be useful against a broad spectrum of species and a wide range of drug resistance mechanisms. Finally, NIH is working with DoD to leverage medical countermeasure programs and resources of mutual interest.

Challenges to Rapidly Expanding the Strategic National Stockpile

Although defining priorities and quantifying the size of the threat to the population are the key steps to focus our efforts, we must be mindful of the realities of the spectrum of efforts needed along the research and development pipeline to produce a useable medical countermeasure. The process of defining required specifications for a countermeasure often reveals few, if any, candidates in the pipeline. Basic research and early development efforts, even when robustly funded, often take years before a concept is mature enough for advanced development. The development of medical products —whether for cancer, influenza, or anthrax – is a complex, lengthy, and expensive process. Ultimate licensure, approval or clearance from FDA requires the rigorous accumulation of sufficient data in humans and animals to establish the safety and efficacy of the product for a specific use and the ability to consistently manufacture the product to meet the appropriate standards. It is important to note that a unique aspect of the pathway for medical countermeasures is the need to establish efficacy either using surrogate markers (such as the human immune response) or, using appropriate animal models, under the "Animal Rule" (*Federal Register* 67:37988-37998, 2002) because demonstration of efficacy against the actual diseases in humans is most often not feasible either because the disease does not occur naturally or for the obvious ethical reasons that prevent exposing humans to the threat agent. The USG is working to provide support for the developers of priority medical countermeasures through the research and development phases, and, when a product has reached the advanced development stage Project BioShield provides an important incentive for manufacturers to take the product the rest of the way through the pipeline. And, as I have outlined here today, in the less than eleven months since Project BioShield was enacted, the incentive has expedited final development of several products for the Stockpile.

Conclusion

In closing, I must emphasize that the number of threat agents against which we could guard ourselves is endless and new and emerging threats introduced by nature or man will present continuing challenges. Although we cannot be prepared for every threat, we have the ability to create a strategic approach to identifying and combating the greatest threats. HHS and its agencies including NIH, CDC, and FDA, have a clear mandate from President Bush and Congress to lead the charge in this arena. We have already made important strides and will continue to work to address the obstacles identified. Mr. Chairman, I look forward to working with you and members of the Subcommittee to address the challenges of bioterrorism preparedness and its impact on public health.

I will be happy to answer any questions you may have.

Mr. MARCHANT [presiding]. Thank you, Mr. Secretary.

The chairman had to attend a Rules Committee meeting and I will be chairing for a while.

At this time, I will recognize Dr. Vitko.

STATEMENT OF JOHN VITKO, JR.

Dr. VITKO. Good afternoon. Thank you very much for inviting me here to speak to you today on DHS's role in this process.

We at DHS do not develop medical countermeasures but play a critical role in informing and guiding the prioritization of those medical countermeasures. I would like to cover four key steps in that process today: threat assessments and determinations conducted specifically to guide Project BioShield, a broader set of risk assessments, a strategy for addressing engineered threats in partnership with and led by the Department of Health and Human Services and scientific studies to better inform these assessments.

As you know, the Project BioShield Act of 2004 charges the Secretary of Homeland Security with the responsibility to determine which biological, chemical, radiological or nuclear threats constitute a material threat to our Nation's security. To fulfill this responsibility, the Department of Homeland Security Science and Technology Directorate, in partnership with our Information Analysis and Infrastructure Protection Directorate, has been conducting formal threat assessments on the agents of greatest concern to establish plausible, high consequence scenarios. These assessments are then used by the Secretary of DHS in determining whether to issue material threat determination and by HHS and the Interagency Weapons of Mass Destruction Medical Countermeasures Subcommittee in determining the need for and the requirements of any new medical countermeasures.

To date, the Secretary of the Department of Homeland Security has issued material threat determinations for four agents: anthrax, smallpox, botulinum toxin and radiological nuclear devices. Additional assessments are underway for plague, tularemia, viral hemorrhagic fevers and chemical nerve agents and will be completed this fiscal year.

DHS has an even broader responsibility in the President's strategy for biodefense for the 21st century. In this strategy, we are charged with conducting formal, periodic risk assessments in coordination with other departments and agencies to guide the prioritization of the Nation's ongoing biodefense activities not just medical but also including such areas as surveillance and detection, decontamination and restoration and forensics.

These risk assessments factor in technical feasibility of a broad range of biological threats. The vulnerability of different portions of our society to those threats and the resulting consequence of any such attacks. The first such formal risk assessment is due in the winter of 2006 and will address all Category A and B agents from the Centers of Disease Control Prevention and Threat List, some Category C agents and a number of potential engineered threats.

Recognizing that the rapid advances in biotechnology demand that we also consider the possibility of engineered threats, we have partnered with HHS and others in formulating and implementing a strategy for anticipating and responding to such threats. Together, we have developed an informed estimate of the types of emerging threats that might be within the ability of a terrorist organization to develop over the near, mid and longer terms and have laid out a strategy for addressing them. The strategy emphasizes ongoing technology watch and risk assessments, rapid surveillance and detection capabilities for engineered threats and expanded range of medical countermeasures and an integrated concept of operations for identifying and responding to emerging or engineered threats.

The threat or risk assessments described above are performed with the best available information. However, there are large uncertainties, sometimes factors of 10 to 100 in some of the key parameters and hence in the associated risks. In one case, it can be the minimum amount of agent needed to infect a person and in another case, it can be the time that such an agent remains viable, that is capable of causing an infection in the air, food or water; and in a third, it can be the effect of food processing or water treatment of the agent's viability.

The Department of Homeland Security has established a National Biodefense Analysis and Countermeasure Center to conduct laboratory experiments needed to close these knowledge gaps. To support this and new facilities being designed and constructed on the National Interagency Biodefense Campus at Fort Detrick, MD. Pending completion of this facility in fiscal year 2008, we have established an interim capability with other Government and private laboratories to begin this vital work.

In summary, the Department of Homeland Security Science and Technology Directorate, in coordination with its Federal partners is conducting a threat and risk assessment critical to prioritizing the Nation's near and long term medical countermeasure development.

This concludes my prepared statement and I would be delighted to answer questions at the appropriate time.

[The prepared statement of Dr. Vitko follows:]

Statement for the Record

Dr. John Vitko, Jr.
Director, Biological Countermeasures Portfolio
Science & Technology Directorate
Department of Homeland Security

Before the U.S. House of Representatives
Committee on Government Reform
Subcommittee on National Security, Emerging Threats,
and International Relations

June 14, 2005

INTRODUCTION

Good afternoon, Chairman Shays, Congressman Kucinich and distinguished members of the Subcommittee. I am pleased to appear before you today to discuss the role that the Department of Homeland Security's (DHS) threat and risk assessments play in informing and prioritizing research and development of new medical countermeasures.

Before focusing on the Department's specific activities in the area of threat and risk assessments, I would like to put these activities in the broader context of the overall responsibilities and activities of the DHS Biological Countermeasures Portfolio (Bio Portfolio) which I direct. The mission of this Portfolio is to provide the understanding, technologies, and systems needed to anticipate, deter, protect against, detect, mitigate, and recover from possible biological attacks on this nation's population, agriculture or infrastructure.

In addressing this mission, DHS has a leadership role in several key areas and partners with lead agencies in others. Those areas in which the Science and Technology (S&T) Directorate provides significant leadership are:

- Providing an overall end-to-end understanding of an integrated biodefense strategy, so as to guide the Secretary and the rest of the Department in its responsibility to coordinate the nation's efforts to deter, detect, and respond to acts of biological terrorism.

- Providing scientific support to better understand both current and future biological threats and their potential impacts so as to guide the research and development of biodefense countermeasures such as vaccines, drugs, detection systems and decontamination technologies.

- Developing early warning, detection and characterization systems to permit timely response to mitigate the consequence of a biological attack.

- Conducting technical forensics to analyze and interpret materials recovered from an attack to support attribution.

- Operation of the Plum Island Animal Disease Center to support both research and development (R&D) and operational response to foreign animal diseases such as foot and mouth disease.

DHS also supports our partnering departments and agencies with their leads in other key areas of an integrated biodefense: the Department of Health and Human Services (HHS) on medical countermeasures and mass casualty response; the Department of Defense (DoD) on broad range of homeland security/homeland defense issues; the U.S. Department of Agriculture (USDA) on agriculture biosecurity; USDA and HHS on food security; the Environmental Protection Agency (EPA) on decontamination and on water security; the Department of Justice on bio-terrorism investigations; and the Intelligence Community on threat warnings.

THREAT AND RISK ASSESSMENTS

As noted above, providing threat and risk assessments of both current and future threats and the scientific understanding to improve and refine these assessments is a major responsibility for DHS. These responsibilities are further defined in the BioShield Act of 2004, which charges the Secretary of DHS with the responsibility for determining which threats constitute a Material Threat to the national security or public health of the Nation and in the President's *Biodefense for the 21st Century,* which charges DHS with the lead in "conducting routine capabilities assessments to guide prioritization of our ongoing investments in biodefense-related research, development, planning and preparedness".

Today, I would like to focus on four major activities that we have undertaken to fulfill these responsibilities:

1. Material Threat Assessments and Determinations in support of Project BioShield;
2. Risk Assessments to guide prioritization of the Nation's ongoing biodefense-related activities;
3. A Strategy for Addressing Emerging Threats (in partnership with the Department of Health and Human Services (DHHS) and others);
4. Scientific research to better inform these threat and risk assessments.

Material Threat Assessments and Determinations for Project BioShield

Working with the DHS Directorate for Information Analysis and Infrastructure Protection (IAIP), DHS S&T has been conducting assessments and determinations of biological, chemical, radiological and nuclear agents of greatest concern so as to guide near-term BioShield requirements and acquisitions. In this process, IAIP, in concert with other members of the intelligence community, provides information on the capabilities, plans and intentions of terrorists and other non-state actors. However, since lack of intelligence on a threat does not mean lack of a threat, S&T, in concert with appropriate members of the technical community, also assesses the technical feasibility of a terrorist being able to obtain, produce and disseminate the agent in question. This information is used to establish a plausible high consequence scenario that provides an indication of the number of exposed individuals, the geographical extent of the exposure, and other collateral effects. If these consequences are of such a magnitude to be of significant concern to our national security or public health, the Secretary of DHS then issues a formal Material Threat Determination to the Secretary of HHS, which initiates the BioShield process.

To date, the Secretary of DHS has issued Material Threat Determinations for four "agents": anthrax, smallpox, botulinum toxin, and radiological/nuclear devices. Additional threat assessments are underway for the remainder of the agents (plague, tularemia, viral hemorrhagic fevers) identified by the Centers for Disease Control and Prevention as Category A agents and for chemical nerve agents. These assessments will be completed this fiscal year.

Once a Material Threat Determination (MTD) has been issued, the HHS then assesses the potential public health consequences of the identified agent and determines the need for countermeasures. After notifying Congress of its determination, HHS evaluates the availability of current countermeasures and the possibility of development of new countermeasures. They are assisted in this by the interagency Weapons of Mass Destruction Medical Countermeasures (WMD-MC) subcommittee of the Office of Science and Technology Policy's National Science and Technology Council (NSTC). The WMD-MC further explores the medical consequences associated with the particular threat and the availability of appropriate countermeasures so as to develop a recommendation for the acquisition of a specific countermeasure. These recommendations then form the basis of the U.S. Government requirements. After approval of these requirements by the Office of Management and Budget, the HHS issues a Request for Proposals and implements and manages the subsequent acquisition process through delivery of the countermeasures to the Strategic National Stockpile.

Risk Assessments to Guide Prioritization of the Nation's Biodefense Activities

The preceding discussion dealt with threat assessments to guide BioShield acquisition processes. DHS has an even broader responsibility in the President's National Biodefense Strategy and that is to conduct formal, periodic risk assessments, in coordination with other Departments and agencies, to guide the prioritization of the nation's ongoing biodefense activities – not just medical, but also including such areas as surveillance and detection, decontamination and restoration, and forensics. These risk assessments provide a systematic look at the technical feasibility of a broad range of biological threats, the vulnerability of different portions of our society to those threats, and the resulting consequences of any such attacks.

The first such formal risk assessment is due in the winter of 2006, with subsequent assessments due every two years. The scope, process and timescale for this first assessment have been presented to and agreed to by the interagency Biodefense Policy Coordinating Committee co-chaired by the Homeland Security Council and the National Security Council. This assessment is addressing:

- All six category A agents from the Centers for Disease Control and Prevention (CDC) threat list;
- All 12 category B agents;
- Five representative category C agents; and
- A number of candidate drug-resistant and emerging agents.

Key outputs will include:

- A list of bio-threats prioritized by risk;
- A prioritized list of critical knowledge gaps that if closed should reduce risk assessment uncertainty and guide bio-defense research and development; and
- A list of biodefense vulnerabilities that could be reduced by countermeasure development and acquisition.

This risk assessment is being conducted in partnership with the Intelligence Community, the HHS, the Department of Defense, the U.S. Department of Agriculture, the Environmental Protection Agency and others. Two advisory boards, one a Government Stakeholders Advisory Board and the other an Independent Risk Assessment Expert Review Board (academia, industry and government) have been established to provide input and advice.

This and subsequent risk assessments will play a critical role in informing future biodefense programs across all agencies, including BioShield acquisitions and the longer-term medical R&D leading up to such acquisitions.

A Strategy for Addressing Emerging Threats

Much of the biodefense efforts to date have focused on protecting against attacks with bioterrorism agents that can be (or used to be) found in nature. However, rapid advances in biotechnology demand that we also consider the possibility and impact of emerging or engineered agents. e.g. modifications to organisms that increase their resistance to medical countermeasure or make them more difficult to detect. The President's *Biodefense for the 21st Century* assigns the HHS the lead in anticipating such future threats. We, DHS S&T, are partnering with HHS and others in formulating and implementing a strategy for anticipating and responding to such threats.

Based on intelligence information, available literature and expert judgment, we have developed an informed estimate of the types of emerging threats that might be within the ability of a terrorist organization to develop over the near (1-3 years), mid (4-10 years), and longer-terms (10 yrs). We have also examined the impact of these threats on the four pillars of the National Biodefense Policy: Threat Awareness, Prevention and Protection, Surveillance and Detection, and Response and Recovery.

In this analysis, four elements stand out as essential to an effective defense against emerging threats:

- Threat, vulnerability and risk assessments to prioritize these threats in terms of the difficulty of their development and deployment, as well as their potential consequences;
- Surveillance and detection capabilities to rapidly detect and characterize engineered agents in environmental and clinical samples so as to provide timely guidance in the selection of the appropriate medical countermeasure;

- An expanded range of safe and effective medical countermeasures and an infrastructure to support rapid research, development, test and evaluation (RDT&E) of new medical countermeasures; and
- integrated concepts of operation (CONOPS) for the identification and response to emerging threats. In addition to conducting these assessments, DHS will continue to collaborate with HHS as it leads efforts to anticipate agents and to facilitate the availability of medical countermeasures.

Scientific research to better inform these threat and risk assessments

The threat and risk assessments described above are performed with the best available information. However, there are large uncertainties, sometimes factors of ten to a hundred, in some of the key parameters and hence in the associated risks. One of the major functions of the threat and risk assessments is to identify these critical knowledge gaps, which can differ for different threat scenarios – in one case it can be the minimum amount of agent needed to infect a person; in another case it can be the time that such an agent remains viable (capable of causing an infection) in the air, food or water; and in a third it can be the effect of food processing or water treatment on the agent's viability. Conducting the laboratory experiments to close the critical knowledge gaps is a primary function of DHS's National Biodefense Analysis and Countermeasures Center (NBACC).

Congress has appropriated a total of $128M for design and construction of NBACC with the necessary biocontainment laboratory space and support infrastructure to conduct these and other experiments. NBACC will be built on the National Interagency Biodefense Campus (NIBC) at Ft. Detrick MD, where its close physical proximity to the DoD's United States Army Medical Research Institute for Infectious Diseases (USAMRIID), the NIH's Integrated Research Facility and the USDA's Foreign Disease-Weed Science Research Unit. NBACC is also collaborating with the Centers for Disease Control and Prevention to further address the critical knowledge gaps. The Record of Decision for NBACC's Final Environmental Impact Statement was signed in January 2005. Design of the facility began in March 2005, with construction scheduled to begin in FY 2006 and be complete by the fourth quarter of FY 2008.

Currently, interim capabilities for both NBACC's biological threat awareness and bioforensic analysis functions have been established with other government and private laboratories to allow vital work in these areas to occur during the NBACC facility's construction.

CONCLUSION

In summary, the DHS Science and Technology Directorate's programs in threat and risk assessment play a critical role in the interagency process to develop medical countermeasures against weapons of mass destruction. These threat and risk assessments are conducted in active collaboration with other Federal departments and agencies and with the appropriate technical experts in the government, academia and the private sector as we collectively seek to reduce the threat of a biological attack against this nation's population, its agriculture and its food supply.

This concludes my prepared statement. With the Committee's permission, I request my formal statement be submitted for the record. Mr. Chairman, Congressman Kucinich , and Members of the Subcommittee, I thank you for the opportunity to appear before you and I will be happy to answer any questions that you may have.

Mr. MARCHANT. Thank you, Dr. Vitko.

I would like to acknowledge that we have been joined at this time by Representative Turner from Ohio, Representative Higgins from New York, and Mr. Van Hollen from Maryland.

At this time, I will recognize Dr. Saldarini.

STATEMENT DR. RONALD J. SALDARINI

Dr. SALDARINI. Good afternoon.

My name is Ronald Saldarini. I am currently a scientific and business consultant to the vaccine and pharmaceutical industry. From 1986 to 1999, I was president of the global vaccine business of American Cyanamid and American Home Products. I am here today as a member of the Committee on Accelerating the Research, Development and Acquisition of Medical Countermeasures Against Biological Warfare Agents which was convened by the Institute of Medicine and the National Research Council. In my remarks this afternoon, I would like to draw attention to the committee's central findings and recommendations.

First, let me note that the committee was convened in response to a congressional mandate and was charged with examining the DOD acquisition process for medical countermeasures to protect against biological warfare agents. We were asked to identify factors that were impeding the DOD acquisition process and to recommend strategies for accelerating the process. Our review was conducted throughout 2003.

The scope of the committee's assessment covered early research and development through Food and Drug Administration approval. We did not examine production and procurement activities, the extent or nature of any biological warfare threat or to assess the value to DOD of developing medical countermeasures compared with pursuing other obligations. We worked from the premise that biological weapons pose a threat to the health of military personnel and that additional FDA approved countermeasures are needed.

Under the best of circumstances, developing new vaccines and drugs is technically and financially challenging. Furthermore, developing biodefense products poses additional scientific, regulatory and ethical challenges because it is not always possible to test efficiency in humans. In our review of DOD's work on medical countermeasures, we have found fragmentation of responsibility and authority, changing strategies that had resulted in lost time and expertise, and a lack of financial commitment adequate to meet the requirements of the program's goals.

The work was part of a program covering both medical and non-medical countermeasures against both chemical and biological warfare threats. Responsibility for centralized oversight of the program, for program planning and budgeting and for operational tasks was distributed across several different chains of command.

We viewed the state of the program as an indication that DOD leaders lacked an adequate grasp of the commitment, time, scientific expertise, organizational structure and financial resources required for success in developing vaccines and drugs. We also saw it as an indication that DOD had not given the task sufficient priority to produce the desired result.

In response, we recommended action in several areas. We first recommended making the DOD program a truly high priority which would include organizational, scientifically knowledgeable leadership, scientific infrastructure improvement and necessary funding to achieve program goals. We recommended accomplishing these changes through the creation in DOD of the Medical Biodefense Agency which would be a new agency with comprehensive responsibility for the research and development program for medical countermeasures against biological warfare agents.

We proposed that this agency consolidate the functions and resources of several existing activities to overcome the competing lines of authority and multiple reporting relationships that the committee had found. In the committee's view, it was essential that the head of this agency have direct authority over budgeting and over the full range of agencies management and operational activities including managing candidate products from the science and technology stage into and through the DOD acquisition system.

The committee also recommended giving the Medical Biodefense Agency responsibility for developing medical countermeasures against infectious diseases. We emphasized the agency should have a highly qualified director with strong experience in vaccine and drug research, development and manufacturing. In addition to strengthening the intramural research and development program, the committee encouraged building a strong extramural program to bring the expertise and creativity of industry and the academic community to the task.

External oversight and accountability for performance were also seen as necessary. The committee recommended an annual, independent, external review by a standing group of experts from academia and the biotechnology and pharmaceutical industries. If DOD were not taking the steps necessary to establish an effective program and make appropriate progress, some or all of the responsibility should as a last resort be transferred from DOD to another appropriate Federal agency.

Finally, the committee also pointed out the need for DOD to work with other Federal agencies and the broader scientific community to address other challenges which would include establishing effective collaborations with academia and industry and reducing administrative and legal barriers to such collaborations, meeting the special regulatory challenges in testing biodefense projects, overcoming current and potential bottlenecks from insufficient access to essential research resources, including specialized laboratory facilities, laboratory animals and ensuring the availability of a well trained work force.

For many years, DOD researchers were among the very few pursuing the development of medical countermeasures against biowarfare agents. Despite the recent upsurge in interest, effort and funding aimed at protecting the civilian population against bioterrorism, the committee saw a need for a continuing and effective DOD program to ensure that unique military needs for battlefield protection receives sufficient attention.

Thanks for the opportunity to testify and I am pleased to answer any questions you have.

[The prepared statement of Dr. Saldarini follows:]

GIVING FULL MEASURE TO COUNTERMEASURES: ADDRESSING PROBLEMS
IN THE DoD PROGRAM TO DEVELOP MEDICAL COUNTERMEASURES
AGAINST BIOLOGICAL WARFARE AGENTS

Statement of

Ronald J. Saldarini, Ph.D.
Scientific Consultant

and

Member, Committee on Accelerating the Research, Development, and Acquisition of
Medical Countermeasures Against Biological Warfare Agents
Institute of Medicine and National Research Council
The National Academies

before the

Subcommittee on National Security, Emerging Threats, and International Relations
Committee on Government Reform
U.S. House of Representatives

June 14, 2005

Good afternoon, Mr. Chairman and members of the Committee. My name is Ronald Saldarini. I am currently a scientific and business consultant to the vaccine and pharmaceutical industry. From 1986 to 1999, I was president of the global vaccine business of American Cyanamid (Lederle Praxis) and American Home Products (Wyeth Lederle). I am here today as a member of the Committee on Accelerating the Research, Development, and Acquisition of Medical Countermeasures Against Biological Warfare Agents of the Institute of Medicine (IOM) and the National Research Council (NRC). The Institute of Medicine and National Research Council are part of the National Academies, chartered by Congress in 1863 to advise the government on matters of science and technology.

The report from which I provide my testimony was the product of a study initiated in 2002 in response to a congressional mandate in the National Defense Authorization Act for Fiscal Year 2002 (P.L. 107-107). Seeking to speed the availability of new medical countermeasures (vaccines, therapeutic drugs, and antitoxins) against biological warfare agents, Congress called for a study to identify new approaches to accelerate the review and approval process for these products and to identify methods for ensuring that new countermeasures will be safe and effective. The specific charge to the study committee called for examining the acquisition process of the Department of Defense (DoD) for drugs and vaccines intended to serve as biowarfare countermeasures. The scope of the committee's assessment included early science and technology development (research and development program elements 6.1, 6.2, 6.3) and advanced development (program elements 6.4, 6.5) through approval and licensure of products by the Food and Drug Administration (FDA). The committee's report *Giving Full Measure to Countermeasures: Addressing Problems in the*

DoD Program to Develop Medical Countermeasures Against Biological Warfare Agents was
released in January 2004.

I want to emphasize that the study did not examine production and procurement
processes for medical countermeasures. Furthermore, the committee was not asked to assess
the nature or extent of any biological warfare threat or to compare the value to DoD of
developing medical countermeasures against biological warfare agents relative to the pursuit
of other obligations. The committee viewed its task as resting on the premise that biological
weapons pose a threat to the health of military personnel, and therefore additional FDA-
licensed medical countermeasures are urgently needed.

THE CONTEXT FOR DEVELOPMENT OF MEDICAL
COUNTERMEASURES

Developing new vaccines and drugs is challenging, both financially and technically.
Estimates of the average cost of bringing a new drug to market have ranged from $110
million to $802 million. As few as one candidate product in 5,000 may reach clinical testing,
and only 20 percent of candidates that begin clinical testing reach licensure. Such estimates
are based primarily on data for new drugs, with few equivalent estimates available for
vaccines and other biologics.

The drug and vaccine development process is also time consuming. One industry estimate
presented to the committee was 7 to 12 years for vaccine development, but experience has
shown that successful completion of clinical testing alone can take as long as 20 years.

Although new techniques are likely to speed the discovery of some candidate
countermeasures, they are unlikely to accelerate some of the most time-consuming parts of
the product development process, including the crucial assessments of a product's safety and

efficacy. Biodefense products pose special scientific, regulatory, and ethical challenges because it is generally unacceptable to expose humans to biowarfare agents to establish the efficacy of medical countermeasures.

Until the late 1990s, federally funded efforts to develop medical biodefense countermeasures were based primarily in DoD. Since the late 1990s, a substantial research effort has emerged within the Department of Health and Human Services, and "Project BioShield" now aims to create financial incentives for the pharmaceutical industry to manufacture and license medical countermeasures. The upsurge in funding and effort aimed at protecting the civilian population against bioterrorism will undoubtedly result in new technologies and products that can also help protect military personnel against biological warfare. Nevertheless, the committee saw a need for a continued DoD program because of a concern that reliance on a program to protect the civilian population may not meet unique military needs for battlefield protection.

COMMITTEE CONCLUSIONS CONCERNING DOD EFFORTS TO DEVELOP MEDICAL COUNTERMEASURES

On the basis of its review, conducted in 2003, the committee concluded that the biodefense efforts of DoD were poorly organized to develop and license vaccines, therapeutic drugs, and antitoxins to protect members of the armed forces against biological warfare agents.

The committee found that DoD's work on medical biodefense countermeasures was part of a program that addresses medical and nonmedical countermeasures against both chemical and biological warfare threats. Responsibility for centralized oversight of the Chemical and Biological Defense Program was assigned to the Assistant to the Secretary of Defense for

Nuclear and Chemical and Biological Defense Programs. However, the operational reality was a fragmented process that put research planning and activities for medical countermeasures under the direction of the Defense Threat Reduction Agency in the Office of the Secretary of Defense, while the execution of those activities (i.e., basic and applied research in a laboratory setting) rested largely with personnel of the U.S. Army Medical Research and Materiel Command, which reports to the Army Surgeon General. Management of the acquisition process for candidate countermeasures that have reached the stage of advanced development was the responsibility of the Joint Program Executive Office for Chemical and Biological Defense, which operates under the direction of Army acquisition officials. The scientific and technical work of product development was being carried out by a variety of private sector firms and integrated through the prime systems contract with DynPort Vaccine Company. Program planning and budgeting were directed from within yet another DoD organization, the Joint Chiefs of Staff.

In addition to the fragmentation of responsibility and authority, the committee found changing strategies that resulted in lost time and expertise and a lack of financial commitment commensurate with the requirements of program goals.

This serious situation existed despite declarations that biological warfare poses a significant threat to the safety and effectiveness of the nation's armed forces, the vaccination of large numbers of military personnel against anthrax and smallpox, a DoD commitment to acquire vaccines against all validated biological warfare threats, and concerns about new bioengineered microbial threats.

The committee concluded that DoD had not given the technically difficult, expensive, and time-consuming task of development and licensure of new biodefense vaccines and therapeutic products sufficient priority to produce the intended results. The disjointed and ineffective management and inadequate funding of DoD's efforts were viewed as clear indications that DoD leaders lacked an adequate grasp of the commitment, time, scientific expertise, organizational structure, and financial resources required for success in developing vaccines and other pharmaceutical products. The committee emphasized that the fragmented half-measures of DoD's effort could not be expected to succeed.

RECOMMENDATIONS FOR ACTION

Improving and accelerating DoD's efforts to develop and license new biodefense vaccines and therapeutic products to protect against present and future biological warfare threats will require strong and creative scientific leadership and a sustained commitment of adequate funding and other resources. Maintaining the status quo in DoD only assures a long, costly, and perhaps fruitless wait for new vaccines and therapeutic products, in the committee's view.

The IOM/NRC committee recommended action in several areas to help make the DoD work on medical countermeasures more effective:

- **Make the Development of Medical Countermeasures a Priority**

To ensure that DoD has an effective research and development program for medical biodefense countermeasures, the committee made the following recommendation: The Secretary of Defense and Congress must make the DoD program for medical biodefense countermeasures a high priority.

If the development of medical countermeasures becomes a priority, the committee identified other changes that would have to follow to establish a sound infrastructure for integrated and comprehensive management of all aspects of the research and development work:

- organizing the program to promote accountability and effective coordination throughout all phases of research, development, and product approval;

- installing scientifically knowledgeable leaders with expertise in the development of vaccines and pharmaceutical products;

- supporting the development of a strong scientific infrastructure; and

- providing the necessary funding to achieve program goals.

• Create a Medical Biodefense Agency in DoD

The committee specifically recommended that Congress should *authorize the creation of the Medical Biodefense Agency*, a new DoD agency responsible for the research and development program for medical countermeasures against biological warfare agents.

As proposed by the committee, this agency would *report directly to the Under Secretary of Defense for Acquisition, Technology, and Logistics*.

The Medical Biodefense Agency should *consolidate the functions and resources of several existing activities*. The competing lines of authority and multiple reporting relationships that the committee found in the DoD system are not adequate. The functions of existing medical biodefense programs, along with their personnel and funding, should be transferred to the new Medical Biodefense Agency. This would include the medical biodefense component of the Chemical and Biological Defense Program, including units within the Army such as the U.S. Army Medical Research Institute of Infectious Diseases (USAMRIID) and related activities in the Defense Advanced Research Projects Agency

(DARPA), as well as the medical biodefense component of the Chemical Biological Medical Systems in the Joint Program Executive Office for Chemical and Biological Defense.

In addition, *the research and development program for medical countermeasures against infectious diseases should also be transferred into the Medical Biodefense Agency.* DoD's programs to develop medical countermeasures against biological warfare agents and against infectious diseases of military significance address similar scientific and technological questions and require closely related expertise and facilities. Also, with concerns about biological warfare threats expanding to include a wider range of naturally occurring and novel biological agents, the line between the two programs is becoming even less distinct and meaningful than it was in the past.

The agency should have *a highly qualified director with strong experience in vaccine and drug research and development and manufacturing, including the rapidly evolving contributions of biotechnology.* It is essential that the agency head have *direct authority over the agency's budgeting and over its full range of management and operational activities,* which should extend from basic research through full-scale production. An organizational approach that creates competing lines of authority and multiple reporting relationships, as the matrix scheme observed by the committee does, is not adequate to address the multiple management and scientific challenges that DoD faces.

Of particular importance is ensuring that the Medical Biodefense Agency has the *authority to manage the transition of candidate products from the science and technology stage into, and their progress through, the DoD acquisition system.* The Medical Biodefense Agency should have the authority to use funds from science and technology accounts (e.g., budget activity 6.3) to support Phase 1 and even Phase 2 clinical trials before a candidate product is subject to acquisition system review.

As proposed by the committee, the Medical Biodefense Agency would rely on *both its intramural research and development program and also build a strong extramural program* to bring the expertise and creativity of industry and the academic community to the task. The agency should focus on meeting unique DoD needs, while ensuring that DoD's program is coordinated with and takes full advantage of related NIH activities.

Based on the scope of DoD's medical biodefense program and the experience of other relevant government agencies and the private sector, *the committee found the DoD program to be underfunded.* Nevertheless, the committee advised that the program should be better focused before any substantial increase in funding occurs. A need for increased funding should be expected if the program successfully expands its extramural research, thus needing to absorb personnel and facility costs currently covered separately in accounts of the military services. Further increases in funding are also likely as products move into later phases of development, which traditionally are more costly. Supplemental funding is also needed for renovation or replacement of the U.S. Army Medical Research Institute of Infectious Diseases (USAMRIID) facility, with its unique animal research resources and specialized laboratory facilities.

The committee was strongly persuaded that creation of the Medical Biodefense Agency would be the most effective means of improving DoD's research and development program for medical biodefense countermeasures. This approach allows for continued DoD control over program priorities, integrated planning and management of all stages in the development of medical biodefense countermeasures, increased visibility of and priority for this work within DoD, increased expertise among the program leadership and managers, enhanced opportunity for coordination with related NIH work on bioterrorism countermeasures, and expanded access to contributions from extramural researchers. At the same time, the committee acknowledged the disruption associated with establishing a new agency and the potential difficulty of attracting a director and agency staff with the necessary qualifications.

- **Establish External Oversight and Accountability for Performance**

To monitor the performance of the DoD research and development program, the committee recommended independent, external review by a standing group of experts from academia and the biotechnology and pharmaceutical industries, with that group's findings reported each year to the Secretary of Defense and the Congress.

The committee found that DoD failed to respond adequately to previous reports with similar recommendations for change. Therefore, as a last resort, if DoD does not take steps necessary to establish an effective program and make appropriate progress within 3 years (as judged by the review group), the committee recommended that all or part of this responsibility should be transferred to an agency responsible for promoting the development of medical countermeasures for bioterrorism defense.

- **Address Other Challenges Related to the Development of Medical Countermeasures**

The committee also recommended that DoD address several other issues, often in collaboration with others, to improve prospects for the successful development and licensure of medical biowarfare countermeasures. In particular, DoD will need to *establish effective collaborations with academia and industry and should reduce barriers to collaboration* posed by complex, cumbersome contracting procedures; the potential instability of government funding; and concerns about potential liability risks.

DoD and other federal agencies will need to *meet special regulatory challenges* because efficacy studies in humans for products intended to protect against potentially lethal pathogens are generally not feasible or ethical. DoD should be part of the extensive research and testing that will be needed to establish the scientific basis for the application of new FDA regulatory guidelines that provide for using animal data for this purpose (the "Animal Efficacy Rule"). The committee also noted the need to ensure sufficient funding for FDA to sustain its added efforts to expedite the testing and review of biodefense products.

Another challenge facing DoD and others is *overcoming current and potential bottlenecks related to research resources*, including specialized laboratory facilities with appropriate biosafety features, facilities to study and house the animals that are essential for this research, and facilities that can produce small supplies of candidate countermeasures in compliance with FDA manufacturing standards.

Finally, DoD should contribute to efforts to *ensure the availability of a well-trained workforce* by defining the capabilities that scientific and technical personnel will need to conduct research and development on medical countermeasures and by aiding in the development and implementation of training programs designed to meet those needs. In addition, DoD should seek to attract and retain a skilled workforce by using available means to offer salaries that are competitive with those in academia and industry.

Thank you for the opportunity to testify. I would be pleased to answer any questions the Committee might have.

Mr. MARCHANT. Thank you, Doctor.

Mr. Platts is with us at this point and we will now begin questions. Mr. Turner and Mr. Platts, do you seek recognition for questions? The Chair recognizes Mr. Turner.

Mr. TURNER. Thank you, Mr. Chairman.

I want to thank Chairman Shays for holding this hearing and continuing his efforts in ensuring that our country is prepared in the area of the terrorist threats that we are facing both in the area of first responders and in the areas of our Federal agencies that have responsibilities for coordinating their efforts as we plan and also restructure our assets to address these threats.

Dr. Klein, in looking at your testimony and in light of the chairman's efforts for us to get an understanding of past and current approaches, how we are being flexible in transforming to meet the risk, at the top of page 3 I see your comparison of the past and current approaches and I get a little confused. The first sentence says, "The current CBRN defense strategy, the current strategy, emphasizes a capabilities-based approach rather than the previous approach which provided greater emphasis on prioritizing threat agents and targeting budgetary resources based on validated intelligence." When you talk about the previous approach, you say the previous approach had a greater emphasis on prioritizing threat agents and targeting budgetary resources based on validated intelligence. If we are going away from that, it sounds to me like we are preparing for things that we know aren't likely to happen and diluting resources from things we know may happen but I am certain that is not what you mean.

Going to the next one, it says "Capabilities-based planning focuses more on how adversaries may challenge us than on whom these adversaries might be." You go on to emphasize the reduction of the dependence on intelligence data. Could you give us your thoughts separate from the testimony that is written here on what that contrast means?

Dr. KLEIN. That is certainly a very good question. If you look at the way the Department of Defense is trying to transform, we are trying to go through a capabilities based approach as opposed to the specific threats. If you look at what we had done in the past, we looked at specific things like anthrax, botulism, what is happening in today's environment is we are now seeing a lot of engineered threats, genetic activities and things which we cannot pursue, for example, vaccines against everything the terrorists might throw at us.

What we are trying to look at is a more broadbased generic approach so rather than saying, for example, that country x is developing a specific toxin be it chemical or biological, we are trying to have a more broadbased approach so that we are not having to rely specifically on intelligence. Hopefully we will be able to respond in a more quick and broad way. Certainly the issues facing our Nation, where civilians are being targeted as well, with our advances in genetic engineering, it is very difficult for us to come up with specific antidotes, pills, vaccines for everything the terrorists might throw at us. So therefore, we are going to a more broadbased approach.

We still need actionable intelligence on how to perform but we are trying to do more on capabilities rather than a specific threat.

Mr. MARCHANT. Mr. Platts, do you seek recognition?

Mr. PLATTS. I apologize for my late arrival and do appreciate the written testimonies. There are a couple questions I would like to address.

Dr. Klein, I think in your testimony you talked about the Joint Vaccine Acquisition Program. I am just trying to get an understanding of the $322 million committed in 1997 and where we are today. Am I understanding correctly that we are talking about fiscal years 2012, 2020 is when we expect to see results from this investment we are making?

Dr. KLEIN. We hope we will see investments earlier. As you probably realize, getting a vaccine licensed is challenging at best. It takes a long time. Certainly HHS and DHS as well as Dr. Fauci have realized we have these challenges.

We are doing now with the animal efficacy rule will let us speed up processes. DOD only uses licensed vaccines, so we have a requirement to go through a long and cumbersome process, but we certainly hope we will have these vaccines available prior to 2020. What I think is really changing our ability to license vaccines will be the animal rule and our understanding of genetic characteristics such as a better understanding of the DNA.

Mr. PLATTS. From a funding standpoint, what are the current projections on the cost, the $322 million we have already invested?

Dr. KLEIN. That is correct. During the building of our 5 year budget from 2006 to 2011, we added an additional $2 billion for our chemical-biological defense program. Probably $80 million of that will be directed toward vaccine development so that we can protect our men and women in uniform. Our mission is somewhat easier than the civilian side where they have a very large age group to be under consideration from infants to the elderly. In our case, we have men and women of very healthy, predictable ages. So we are optimistic that some of our applications will come out earlier than those that will be more broadbased for the entire population but we are investing a considerable amount of money for vaccine development.

Mr. PLATTS. The $322 million investment is not a lost investment, that is laying a foundation?

Dr. KLEIN. Yes, it is laying a foundation. It is absolutely not a lost investment. We had clinical trials, we had product development. So it was not money wasted by any means.

Mr. PLATTS. I chair the Subcommittee on Financial Accountability so I am always looking at what we are investing, how we are investing and bottom line, what return are the taxpayers getting, so I understand this is a very complex process and it is multiyear, but I want to make sure that we are moving in the right direction.

Dr. Fauci, on the actual investments or the research being done, how are we not competing with the private sector for the free market reasons for pursuing these projects with tax dollars? How are we guarding against that?

Dr. FAUCI. Actually, we don't want to compete, we want to totally synergize with them. We cannot make countermeasures ourselves. We are not manufacturers of countermeasures. We do the basic research and the clinical and applied research and partner with either biotech or pharmaceutical companies to ultimately develop a countermeasure.

In fact, that is the whole purpose of the BioShield Project where the HHS in the form of NIH predominantly does the research that does the concept development, does the early Phase I, II and sometimes into more advanced development and then the companies partner with us to actually manufacture it and make the commitment which under the circumstances that we have now are being aided by the set aside money, the $5.6 billion in BioShield, to be able to then make a procurement of that. It really is a partnership. It is not at all a competition.

Mr. PLATTS. Thank you.

Mr. MARCHANT. Dr. Klein, in your testimony, you talk about the DOD Clinical and Biological Defense Program activities and state they are informally coordinated with the Department of Health and Human Services. Can you talk to us about the informal agreement and how it works?

Dr. KLEIN. One of the things we do is we have a lot of interaction at the working level where the staff of the Department of Defense meets with Stewart Simonson's staff. We have a lot of technical exchanges, a lot of regular meetings scheduled and in addition, Mr. Simonson and I meet periodically to prioritize to make sure we are spending the taxpayers' dollars in the most effective way, that we are not duplicating.

The current agreement we are trying to work between the two departments is where DOD's role and responsibility will be clearly defined on some of the screening and up to Phase 1, then we will transfer that work through the Department of HHS where they can take it through more of the clinical trials where they have greater expertise than DOD. So we are trying to utilize the expertise of both departments to the benefit of the taxpayer.

Mr. MARCHANT. What steps has DOD taken to respond to the Institute of Medicine?

Dr. KLEIN. We have taken several steps. I was confirmed in 2001 about the time a lot of activities were increasing, obviously the terrorist attack and subsequently the anthrax attacks. We have reorganized the Chemical and Biological Defense Program to have a Joint Requirements Office through the joint staff where they define our requirements; we have organized our science and technology development through the Defense Threat Reduction Agency; we have increased the technical competency of our staff where we have several professional medical staffs onboard; the Deputy for the Chemical and Biological Defense Program is a medical doctor, a former Assistant Surgeon General of the Air Force. We have taken a lot of the recommendations of the Institute of Medicine.

Since then BioShield has been created in addition to the Department of Homeland Security. So there is a lot of activities created since the Institute of Medicine study.

Mr. MARCHANT. Can you explain why the JVAP program should continue to receive funding in its present form?

Dr. KLEIN. The JVAP Program is one which like all programs, it has successes, it has things we would like to occur at a more rapid rate but the program is responsible for the vaccine procurement as well as a lot of the science and technological development. Again we are focusing a lot of attention on that program. The Army is the executive agent for this activity. We have a joint program activity through the Army to coordinate those activities. So we are focusing our attention to hopefully increase the end result and that is to protect our men and women in uniform.

Mr. MARCHANT. Secretary Simonson, you say in your testimony that HHS has defined a three stage development and acquisition strategy with open competition awards at each stage. How are you reaching out to companies who have developed or are in the process of developing countermeasures?

Mr. SIMONSON. That is an important part of the operation of Bio-Shield and our success I think will be contingent upon how well we are out there probing the market to bring firms in to propose on our various projects. One we do it is with request for information where we will actually send out a circular seeking sources to find out what is out there, what companies are making product or investing in products that might be useful to us. It is a way of doing market research and also assessing the state of science.

We are also working very aggressively through the WMD Subcommittee to understand what is going on in other agencies. Dr. Klein mentioned the informal work that he and I are doing to bring our two agencies together. There is also a more formal process, this Weapons of Mass Destruction Subcommittee where you have all of the stakeholders in the Federal research community. That is a place where we can exchange information on who is funding what and try to elicit support for or interest in the projects we are trying to develop.

I think those are two ways that we do it. We are also still learning. There are other ways of reaching out to industry, especially the smaller, biotech companies to keep them interested in Bio-Shield.

Mr. MARCHANT. Do you feel there is sufficient interest out in the biotech industry to try to address these issues? Do you think there is sufficient interest in that industry to stimulate the kind of research we probably need?

Mr. SIMONSON. I think there is sufficient interest. I think the interest is more in the smaller biotech firms than it is in big pharma simply because of the tradeoffs that have to be made. Dr. Fauci talks about the relative tradeoff of cholesterol lowering agent as opposed to a biomedical countermeasure. There is no comparison. The whole vaccine market worldwide is less than one cholesterol lowering agent, so it is not as appealing to the big manufacturers so I think our future is with the small to medium sized biotech firms.

There is a lot of work to bring this along but once you do, you are building an infrastructure, building something within the United States that can be useful to us in other ways. It is a very labor intensive and collaborative process between us and these biotechs. The ultimate result is one that makes the industrial base better in the United States, we think. We saw this with the company that produced the second generation smallpox vaccine.

Mr. MARCHANT. Dr. Saldarini, your committee concluded biodefense efforts of DOD were poorly organized to develop and license vaccines, therapeutic drugs, and antitoxins to protect members of the armed forces against biological warfare agents. What can we expect from the JVAP Program it continues in its current form without implementing your committee's recommendations?

Dr. SALDARINI. First, while JVAP was the topic of conversation during the committee's deliberation, and while it was clear there were some issues with JVAP in terms of their activities for acquisition, it was the committee's conclusion that JVAP was not the sole source of the problem, in fact was a part of a larger problem where it was unclear who was in charge of the program and assessing priorities and how the entire thing was organized to get something done.

If you look at the charts that we looked at as we tried to evaluate the different groups involved, it became very, very difficult to understand the distinction between each of these groups. It was an alphabet soup of acronyms for an outsider who doesn't live in the military or the DOD on a daily basis. It was very difficult to assess who was in charge of what and how things actually got done and how priorities were moved through the systems.

So where JVAP did have some problems, JVAP was not the sole source of the problem. From our perspective, it was the overall organization with an inadequate priority infrastructure funding resource base that created the problem.

This committee finished its activities in 2003, so it has been 18 months since we last, or certainly I looked at it and I don't believe any other of the former committee members have looked at it, so I don't know really what has transpired. There were changes. Apparently Dr. Klein mentioned something about changes with JVAP but I don't know what they are and I don't think any of our committee members do.

We reported what we found at the time. Perhaps things have been streamlined but it is still unclear to me whether or not there is adequate authority available to make things happen in a committee fashion.

Mr. MARCHANT. Thank you.

The committee counsel would like to ask some questions.

Mr. HALLORAN. First, Dr. Fauci, NIAID awarded a grant to the Dynport Vaccine Co. which is the prime integrator or contractor for the Joint Vaccine Acquisition Program. Could you tell us something about that grant and why it looked on the face to be a duplication of paying for an activity that JVAP is already being paid for.

Dr. FAUCI. It may appear that way but it actually is complementary. The grant that we are talking about was actually three grants and a contract to Dynport and the total was I think about $29 million. Two grants were to support development of a vaccine candidate for botulism toxin that complemented the activity that was going on in the Department of Defense.

In addition, there was a grant for Phase II trial of the Venezuelan Equine Encephalitis. Again, although the DOD was also working on that, it was complementary and one was to support research on a vaccine candidate for tularemia which the DOD had responsibility for before but then handed that over to us and we are now working fundamentally on the tularemia.

So if you look at the organisms and match them, you say, wait a minute, the DOD is really doing that but actually in one of them, they are no longer doing the tularemia and the other two are complementary working on aspects of it that the DOD is not.

Mr. HALLORAN. Complementary in the sense of adding the population to the testing profile that Dr. Klein mentioned that the DOD doesn't have to cover?

Dr. FAUCI. There are two things, different scientific aspects but importantly geared toward and Dr. Klein mentioned this in his oral testimony, that they are fundamentally looking at forced protection and the warfighting individuals where we are looking at everything from children up through and including the elderly. It is much more for the civilian population, so a lot of the complementariness is due to the broader scope of people that we are responsible for in the civilian population.

Dr. KLEIN. I think this is an example of the two departments working together very well where we complement to the benefit of the taxpayer rather than duplicate. When you look at just the headlines and don't dig into the technical aspects of it, one can see on paper it might have been duplication until you really look at the details.

Mr. HALLORAN. Why did DOD hand over the tularemia work? Is that not a force protection threat?

Dr. KLEIN. We felt that NIAID had better technical expertise than the Department of Defense. We took it up to a certain point and felt their technical expertise was better than ours.

Mr. HALLORAN. Let us talk about botulism, where we are. The next panel has some testimony about some kind of halting and stumbling attempts to get botulism antitoxin, particularly outside the A and B serotypes. Where are we in that, both in terms of what we have in hand should an attack take place in the United States now or in the military theater and what is coming down the pipeline and when?

Dr. FAUCI. Botulism is a complex issue and is somewhat problematic for a number of reasons that I will briefly describe. There are seven, it is a heptavalent toxin and we are in the process now of making monoclonal antibodies which are antibodies against a particular component of a botulism toxin. The most common that are used are A, B and E but you really have to have sort of a cocktail of all of them.

The difficulty that we face with transitioning from the horse sera botulism antitoxin which has been the standard that has been used both in the unusual occurrence of situations of natural infection with botulism in this country as well as what the DOD has been working on for years as a countermeasure for force protection. The transition from the polyclonal sera and plasma from the horses is taking a lot of time for the simple reason that relates to one of the things we have been saying in one way or another among all of us, the difficulty in engaging researchers and industry on the outside to get involved.

We have one very good researcher that is superb at developing the initial monoclonal antibodies against the individual subtypes of botulism. The difficulty is that this is one group working alone so it takes about 6 months per subtype and then you hand it over to the more industrial related ones that go on do the actual manufacture and the clinical trial.

So if you stagger them at 6 month periods, by the time we get a robust heptavalent polyclonal cocktail, it is going to take several years. It would be wonderful if we had 20 or 30 investigators on it but there just is not the interest that we would like to see for the reasons that people want to work on other things. That gets back to the principle of trying to incentivize not only individual investigators but also companies to get involved.

Right now in an emergency we would have to rely on the polyclonal serum that we have had and are making more of but hopefully we will transition over to the monoclonal antibodies.

Dr. KLEIN. One of the areas and what I am hoping is as we get a better understanding of our DNA structure, that the kinds of research activities that individuals are currently performing will be enhanced by genetic splicing, DNA splicing and things of that nature. So we are hopeful that we will be able to get products out quicker with our understanding of the basic fundamental responses under our DNA.

Dr. SALDARINI. I can talk about the current generation botulinum program. HHS picked up after September 11th a DOD program that began during the first Gulf war to hyperbenize horses against all seven serotypes and then to ferrice them and collect this hyperimmune plasma but it was never finished. They just had fairly substantial amount of hyperimmune plasma in storage. It was transferred to us I think at the end of 2002.

HHS undertook to have that material processed. This was a process that hasn't been done in an awful long time, so the firm we engaged to do it had to spend a lot of time moving deliberately because of the risk of losing material if they made a mistake. In any event, that work is done. They finished processing the plasma. We had sort of mixed results on the yield because of the age of the plasma and so forth. I would be happy to come to your office give you more detail on exactly how much we have. We don't talk about it openly.

We also have a program now where a whole new population of horses is being hyperimmunized against all seven serotypes. This is an example of where things can't be rushed beyond what science will allow. The horses have been immunized and then challenged with botulinum but it takes a period of time to get the titer up so you can actually begin to ferrice them.

We expect some time in the fall that we will have enough hyperimmune plasma that we can begin processing the new material. We have an objective, an ultimate objective of 100,000 treatment courses of heptavalent antitoxin but it is a big operation, 200 horses over a few farms and it is also I have learned as much an art as it is a science.

The current botulinum toxoid or vaccine is no longer licensed, it is in IND status and there is a cohort within the research community and at the Defense Department that has a need for botulinum vaccine and so we are looking at what options are available there.

Dr. VITKO. It is an interesting term because I use capabilities with a slightly different meaning. Right now I believe that it still makes a lot of sense to look agent by agent in terms of the extent of the threat that they pose. So we look at the feasibility of a terrorist organization engineering that threat, producing that agent, disseminating it and look at the consequences associated with it and we do make use of intelligence information both on interest by known organizations, skills levels associated with those organizations to give some assessment of what could be done, but then we really do take a look at the scientific basis for producing that agent and disseminating it, irrespective of the threat group. We believe at this stage that is the best way of assessing what constitutes a material threat to this country. Material threat determination says if an organization can produce it, is it one. As you heard, we postulated and formulated working with HHS in an interagency forum a timeline for when we think certain engineered threats could come on and the general characteristics of those. We have developed a strategy for dealing with that as well as a hedge strategy in case our projections are off.

I think in that sense it will be a while until we get to the goal where we can treat broad classes of agents as a class and until we have, as desirable as it is, sort of broadbased either vaccines or antibiotics for dealing with those. That doesn't take away from that being a desirable R&D goal but for near term strategy, I think it does have to focus on which agents pose the greatest risk in the current scenarios.

Mr. HALLORAN. Thank you.

Mr. MARCHANT. The Chair acknowledges that Mr. Duncan from Tennessee has joined us. Mr. Duncan, do you have any questions?

Mr. DUNCAN. Thank you and since I just got here, I won't ask any questions but I will say this. I am disturbed about this statement or Chairman Shays' that says "A 2004 study by the Institute of Medicine found that the Department of Defense Biodefense Program fragmented and often prey to competing priorities. Launched in 1997 with $322 million, the JVAP has spent that much and more. Yet lists of JVAP accomplishments provided to the subcommittee included just one recently licensed therapeutic, no completed vaccines and two target vaccine programs terminated after significant expenditures."

I notice there is testimony from one of the witnesses on the next panel that says "This procurement process which formally began on April 1, 2004 and has yet to be completed 14 months later is simply too long and too burdensome to sustain continued interest in participating in BioShield by companies such as Human Genome Sciences whose principal focus is not the Federal sector."

I serve on three different committees and several different subcommittees and I read articles and columns all the time about what all these other committees and subcommittees do. It seems that every day we see examples of unbelievable waste and inefficiency here at the Federal level. It seems if we want something to cost 10 or 15 times more than it should and 10 or 15 times more than it would with fewer results than if the private sector did it or if State and local governments did it, just turn it over to the Federal Government. It gets pretty tiresome to hear this out of every department and agency.

Everybody today, because we have a patriotic fervor going on wants to give the Department of Defense everything they ask for and more but the waste and inefficiency, we had a hearing in this committee last week which said the Department of Defense has blown $466 million in its ordinary procurement processes. We just gloss over things like that because I guess figures in the billions and $466 million are too big to comprehend but it gets pretty sad after a while.

Thank you, Mr. Chairman.

Mr. MARCHANT. Thank you, Mr. Duncan.

I thank the panel today for its participation and we will recognize the next panel. Our next panel will be: Dr. Michael G. Hanna, Jr., Chief Scientific Officer, Intracel and Dr. James H. Davis, executive vice president and general counsel, Human Genome Sciences, Inc.

[Witnesses sworn.]

Mr. MARCHANT. At this time, the Chair will recognize Dr. Hanna for his testimony.

STATEMENTS OF DR. MICHAEL G. HANNA, JR., CHIEF SCIENTIFIC OFFICER, INTRACEL; AND DR. JAMES H. DAVIS, EXECUTIVE VICE PRESIDENT AND GENERAL COUNSEL, HUMAN GENOME SCIENCES, INC.

STATEMENT OF DR. MICHAEL G. HANNA, JR.

Dr. HANNA. First of all, let me say how grateful I am for having the opportunity to address this congressional committee. As you, I am also concerned that such a committee meeting on the Elusive Antidotes of CBRN Countermeasures must be held in June 2005.

I would like to tell you about a successful development of a unique therapy for botulinum toxin exposure. This story consists of scientific success and extreme frustration. There are seven serotypes of botulinum toxin. They have been identified as the most dangerous biological substances and the most likely biological weapons of mass destruction.

The success is that my company, Intracel, through a Department of Defense contract, referred to earlier by one of you, between 1991 and 1996 was successfully able to develop a heptavalent equine antibody product that was efficacious in combating the seven serotypes of botulinum toxin, was safe in humans and was FDA-approved for emergency use. We made 5,000 therapeutic doses before the project was terminated by the Joint Program Office of the Department of Defense in 1996. It was terminated at this point because we had proof of principle and a botulinum crisis was improbable. Since September 11th, however, the improbable became probable.

Today, Federal officials fear the world is vulnerable to such an attack and we are ill prepared if one were to occur. In fact, Tommy Thompson in his exit speech to HHS declared that he was surprised that such an attack had not already occurred, which also surprised me that he would say that. Dr. Anthony Fauci of NIAID was quoted that this is one of the Federal Government's top bioterrorism interests and "we are marshaling all available resources." This statement was made in 2002; yet as far as I know, as of last year, we still had only the residual several thousand therapeutic doses left over from Intracel's previous effort. Today there was some discussion where they were not prepared to discuss what they have today generated from the new contract and I can tell you they have monoclonal product only not heptavalent product.

I was at a meeting with the Department of Defense, the Army, when one of them mentioned that they had monoclonals to A and B and Congressman Dr. Roscoe Bartlett said, let us not let the terrorists know that because then all they have to worry about is C through G.

This is my frustration. With our scientific success of overcoming the hurdles to produce such an important therapeutic product, we have not been successful in fulfilling our destiny of producing the hundreds of thousands of doses necessary to protect our military and civilian populations at risk. In Los Angeles, they had a simulated botulism attack which was very successfully carried out. They calculated they would have needed 600,000 doses to protect the population at risk. This was months ago. We are no where close to having that number of therapeutic doses.

The NIH used considerable resources to fund grants to make recombinant vaccines for protection of botulinum infection and to develop drugs which would interfere with the enzymatic activity of the organism. These efforts however worthwhile are problematic 10 year endeavors.

Today, Intracel holds the intellectual property, over 300 standard operating procedures and all the necessary equipment to produce the proven heptavalent equine therapeutic product and was willing and capable of generating through private funds to develop a subsidiary that would build a validated manufacturing facility and produce 50,000 therapeutic doses in 2 years. The yield would be more than 100,000 doses per year thereafter. We made this proposal in 2002.

In addition, using our own moneys, Intracel offered to complete the research program and begin the next generation product using safer and more effective human monoclonal antibodies. We happen to be the only company that has ever made a licensed human monoclonal antibody. This second generation product could be prophylactically used and be safe for multiple injections for better protection of the troops after an exposure.

Clearly, we thought we were the poster child of BioShield. However, in spite of who we contacted and how hard we tried, we could not get the Government to give us a written commitment to purchase the product based on our success in meeting the specifications that we had established for the DOD in 1997. We talked to everybody and anybody and we had Congressman Shays and Congressman Bartlett with us at many of the meetings.

It seems that the Government agencies are not really marshaling efforts to deal with this problem. The agencies have relegated down to the ranks of the functionaries and contract and grants sections and if they have the urgency that this issue requires, it has not overcome the status quo.

I would like to know what we would have done last year, this year or next year if such a botulinum toxic weapon was used in the United States in the real sense, not in a simulated sense as we did in Los Angeles a few months ago. Clearly the BioShield concept with all of its good intentions has not gained the strength to overcome the status quo.

I would like to repeat, Intracel was not asking the Government to pay for the production of this important component of our medical armament for biodefense. Intracel was asking the Government to give us a commitment to buy the product if we met specifications already paid for by the Department of Defense. That probably was our mistake in not asking for money.

To rapidly generate required antidotes and therapies for weapons of mass destruction requires a paradigm of built-in redundancies such as those employed in successful NASA goals and accomplishments after the Presidential mandate by President Kennedy. I would have thought that BioShield provided the capability to build in redundancies but it appears to me from people I have talked to, BioShield does not impart this kind of legislation.

Thus, I recommend to this subcommittee that the BioShield legislation should be rewritten so that it funds multiple groups and creates competition of several companies up to Phase 1 trials, then let the survivor of the most competent prevail. With that type of competitions, you would have redundancies to better guarantee success and you can end up with the stockpiles that will save lives if such an emergency occurs. No longer should we rely on these products being generated by the low bidders as an independent agent for any agency.

Second, I think what we saw this morning is that the stovepipe type of funding coming down through the agencies does not really bode well for interagency interactions which we are going to need both at the development level, the manufacturing level and mostly at the level of preparedness and defense out in the field, the States and the counties and the cities if such an attack ever occurs.

Thank you.

[The prepared statement of Dr. Hanna follows:]

Presentation to Congressional Subcommittee on
National Security, Emerging Threats, and International Relations
June 14, 2005
Michael G. Hanna, Jr.
Chairman (Emeritus) and Chief Scientific Officer
Intracel

First of all let me say how grateful I am for having the opportunity to address this Congressional committee. I am also concerned that such a committee meeting on the "Elusive Antidotes of CBRN Countermeasures" must be held in June of 2005. Before I begin my formal presentation I would like to emphasize to the committee that besides my training in immunology and scientific success in developing immunotherapeutic approaches to treating cancer and infectious diseases, I have been a volunteer on federal, state and county committees for Homeland Security. From 1984 to 1989 I directed the commerce departments Biotechnology Advisory Committee, and recently directed the Frederick County Local Emergency Planning Committee responsible for Weapons of Mass Destruction threat assessment, preparedness and response.

I would like to tell you about the successful development of a unique therapy for Botulinum toxin exposure, which consists of scientific success and frustration. The seven serotypes of botulinum toxin have been identified as the most dangerous biological substances and the most likely biological weapon of mass destruction. The success is that my company Intracel, through a DoD contract between 1991 and 1996 was able to successfully develop a heptavalent equine antibody product that was efficacious in combating the seven serotypes of Botulinum toxin, was safe in humans and was FDA approved for emergency use. We made 5000 therapeutic doses before the project was terminated by the JPO in 1996. It was terminated at this point because we had proof of principal and a Botulinum crises was improbable. Since 9/11 however the improbable became probable.

Today, Federal officials fear the world is vulnerable to such an attack and that we are ill prepared if one were to occur. In fact, Tommy Thompson in his exit speech declared that he was surprised that such an attack had not already occurred. Dr. Anthony Fauci of the NIH/NIAID is quoted as pointing out that this is one of the Federal governments top bioterrorism interests, and we are "marshalling all available resources". This statement was made in 2002, yet as far as I know as of last year we still only had the residual 3000 therapeutic doses left over from Intracel's previous effort.

This is my frustration. We have been successful in overcoming the scientific hurdles to produce this important therapeutic product; however, we have not been successful in fulfilling our destiny of producing the hundreds of thousands of doses necessary to protect our military and civilian populations at risk.

The NIH has used considerable resources to fund grants to make recombinant vaccines for protection of Botulinum infection and to develop drugs which would interfere with the enzymatic activity of the organism. These efforts, however, worthwhile are problematic, 10 year endeavors. Intracel holds the intellectual property, over 300 standard operating procedures and all of the necessary equipment to produce the proven, heptavalent equine therapeutic product and was willing and capable of generating private funds to develop a subsidiary that would build a validated manufacturing facility and produce 50,000 therapeutic doses in 2 years. The yield would be 100,000 or more doses each year thereafter. Clearly, we thought we were the poster child of Bioshield. However, we could not get the government to give us a written commitment to purchase the product based on our success in meeting their expectations.

The CDC, the agency responsible for developing this product since the late 1990s, did finally approve a contract with a foreign company to make heptavalent equine Botulism antitoxin. As of last year, they had not generated any therapeutic doses. In 2002 we were contacted by a senior member of NIH/NIAID (Dr. Dennis Lang) who asked us to generate a grant proposal which would fund Intracel to produce the product. Although I questioned this approach, I did comply but the grant was turned down due to the NIH "color of money". The embarrassed NIH officers then encouraged me to submit an unsolicited proposal to the CDC, which I did, and this too was turned down. At the same time I visited several congressmen and directors of responsible DoD and NIH research laboratories, and Congressman Shays shared this experience through a letter to the directors of HHS and DHS. No letter of commitment was forthcoming; in fact many of them claimed that they did not have the authority to make a commitment. This was very frustrating and we finally gave up.

It seems to me that the government agencies are not really marshalling its efforts to deal with this problem. The agencies have relegated down the ranks to the contract and grants people. If they have the urgency of the matter, it has not overcome the status quo. In fact, much of the money has been devoted to basic research at the expense of the less problematic, pragmatic approach.

I would like to know what we would have done last year, or this year or next year if such a botulinum toxin weapon was used in the US. Clearly, the Bioshield concept with all of its good intentions has not gained the strength to overcome the status quo. I would like to repeat, Intracel was not asking the government to pay for the production of this important component of our medical armamentarium for Biodefense, Intracel was asking the government to give us a commitment to buy the product if it met specifications already paid for by the DoD.

Thank you for listening.

Mr. MARCHANT. Thank you, Dr. Hanna.
Dr. Davis.

STATEMENT OF JAMES H. DAVIS

Dr. DAVIS. Mr. Chairman, members of the subcommittee, thank you for the invitation to appear before you today on behalf of Human Genome Sciences.

I am Jim Davis, executive vice president and general counsel of HGS. In this capacity I have been extensively involved with the business development, regulatory approval process and Federal procurement issues related to the anticipated sale of our innovative, therapeutic treatment Abthrax for victims of anthrax exposure. We undertook this project on our own initiative and at our own expense.

HGS is a biopharmaceutical company located in nearby Rockville, MD that discovers, develops and manufactures innovative drugs to treat and cure disease. Currently, we have seven drugs including Abthrax in clinical development, including six monoclonal antibodies.

The primary focus of our company, however, is not the development of drugs to protect against attack by biological and chemical weapons. The principal focus of our company has been and will continue to be pursuit of innovative biopharmaceutical products for the commercial market. Nevertheless, just over 3 years ago we realized that our company had significant technology and capability to develop an effective, near term countermeasure against one of the Nation's most immediate and serious bioterrorism threats.

Located just outside Washington, DC, we witnessed firsthand the potentially devastating effects of the use of anthrax as a terrorist weapon in late 2001. Using our own funds, we developed a fully human monoclonal antibody drug called Abthrax that can prevent and treat the lethal effects of anthrax infection. The drug can be given prior to or after exposure, can be used alone or in conjunction with the current vaccine and antibiotics.

We have shown in animals that it is effective against high doses of anthrax, we have demonstrated initial safety in humans and we have been ready to manufacture this product and complete the final human safety trials for over a year and a half, but to move forward we need to bring to conclusion the lengthy procurement process now underway with the Federal Government.

If a contract is signed with the Federal Government and a final commitment to acquire a fixed number of doses and the number of doses requested is of sufficient commercial quantity to make it worthwhile, this countermeasure could be available for emergency use as early as next year. While this is an exciting prospect for our company and of valuable benefit to the Nation, our frustration remains the Federal Government could have had this product in the stockpile already if the full authority of Project BioShield had been used as intended.

The primary challenge of biopharmaceutical companies such as HGS in this field is the absence of a commercial market for bioterrorism countermeasures. The only valuable market is the Federal Government and perhaps our foreign allies. Without a clear and easily accessible market, the drug will not be developed.

In its initial BioShield solicitation for anthrax therapies, HHS has not even specified the precise amount of quantity they wish to purchase. Rather, the solicitation requires bidders to pose pricing for a broad range of quantities ranging from 10,000 doses to 200,000 doses. It now appears that even if this contract is awarded and HHS decides to exercise its option for the manufacture, HHS is unlikely to purchase a full 200,000 doses as originally proposed.

This is particularly frustrating since the manufacture of these compounds requires significant manufacturing capability and significant manufacturing startup costs. In short, the cost per dose of 200,000 doses is significantly less than the cost of 100,000 doses and astronomically less than the amount for 10,000 doses.

Setting a firm commitment for the quantity to be purchased and making sure those quantities are large enough to be commercially viable is critical to advance BioShield's purpose of promoting the development of a biodefense industry.

My written testimony raises additional concerns. There are several steps HHS could undertake to increase industry participation. In the interest of time, I will not enumerate them here. Let me say, however, that timing is critical. I applaud the subcommittee for its continued oversight of this critical biodefense program. Near term delays in evaluating and considering the production of viable countermeasures can disproportionately prolong the procurement of such drugs. To date, abthrax has been developed entirely with private funds but to move forward, we need a firm commitment from the Government to purchase this product. With sufficient Government support, HGS could begin producing significant quantities of Abthrax by the end of next year.

We look forward to formalizing this commitment in a contract with HHS in the coming weeks and we would appreciate every effort to ensure that maximum quantities are purchased for the stockpile as soon as possible without any further delay.

Thank you for this opportunity to testify and I look forward to answering your questions.

[The prepared statement of Dr. Davis follows:]

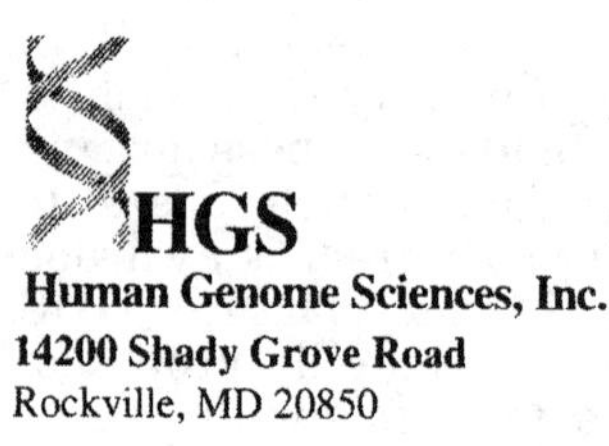

Human Genome Sciences, Inc.
14200 Shady Grove Road
Rockville, MD 20850

Testimony of
James H. Davis, Ph.D.
Executive Vice President and General Counsel
Human Genome Sciences, Inc.
Before the United States House of Representatives
Committee on Government Reform,
Subcommittee on National Security, Emerging Threats, and
International Relations

June 14, 2005

Hearing on "State of BioDefense in the United States"

Mr. Chairman, members of the Subcommittee, thank you for the invitation to appear before you today on behalf of Human Genome Sciences. I am Dr. Jim Davis, Executive Vice President and General Counsel of Human Genome Sciences. In this capacity, I have been extensively involved with the business development, regulatory approval process, and federal procurement issues related to the anticipated sale of Human Genome Sciences' innovative therapeutic treatment, ABthrax, for victims of anthrax exposure. I have been involved with this project since we undertook to develop this product on our own initiative and at our own expense immediately following the anthrax attacks of 2001.

Human Genome Sciences is a biopharmaceutical company located in Rockville, Maryland, that discovers, develops and manufactures gene-based drugs to treat and cure disease. Currently, we have seven drugs in clinical development, including six monoclonal antibodies,

- 2 -

and a broad pipeline of preclinical compounds. These include novel human protein and antibody drugs discovered through our genomics-based research, as well as new, improved, long-acting versions of existing proteins created using our albumin fusion technology.

ABthrax™

Let me be clear. The primary focus of Human Genome Sciences has *not* been the development of drugs to protect against attack by biological and chemical weapons. The principal focus of our company has been, and remains, pursuit of innovative bio-pharma products for the commercial market. We are not a "bio-defense" company as that term has come to be known in the post-9/11 environment. Our business plan, our executives, and our investors do not see the primary focus of Human Genome Sciences, now or in the future, to be the federal market place.

Nevertheless, just over three years ago, we realized that our company had the technology and capability to develop an effective, near-term countermeasure against one of the nation's most immediate and serious bioterrorism threats – anthrax. As a company headquartered just outside Washington D.C., we witnessed first-hand the potentially devastating effects of the use of anthrax as a terrorist weapon in late 2001. Thus, using our own funds, Human Genome Sciences developed a fully human monoclonal antibody drug – called ABthrax – that specifically binds to a key anthrax toxin, thereby preventing or treating the lethal effects of anthrax infection.

The drug can be given prior to or after exposure; and it could be used alone or in conjunction with the current vaccine and antibiotics. We have shown, in animals, that ABthrax is effective against high doses of anthrax, and have demonstrated initial safety in humans, and have been ready to begin manufacturing of this product and to initiate additional human safety trials for over a year and a half. In order to move forward, however, we need to bring to a favorable conclusion the lengthy procurement process now underway for the federal government to enter into a contract under the Project Bioshield Act of 2005 to purchase the drug for the Strategic National Stockpile. Once this contract is signed, this key biodefense countermeasure could be available for emergency use as early as next year. While this is an exciting prospect for our company – and a valuable benefit to the Nation – our frustration remains that the federal

- 3 -

government could have had this product in the Strategic National Stockpile already if the full authority of Project Bioshield been used as intended.

As you know, anthrax infection is caused by a spore-forming bacterium, *Bacillus anthracis,* which multiplies in the body and produces lethal toxins. Most anthrax fatalities are caused by the irreversible effects of the anthrax toxins. Research has shown that protective antigen is the key facilitator in the progression of anthrax infection at the cellular level. After protective antigen and the other anthrax toxins are produced by the bacteria, protective antigen binds to the anthrax toxin receptor on cell surfaces and forms a protein-receptor complex that makes it possible for the anthrax toxins to enter the cells. Human Genome Sciences' ABthrax antibody blocks the binding of protective antigen to cell surfaces and prevents the anthrax toxins from entering and killing the cells.

Currently, two options are available for the prevention or treatment of anthrax infections – a vaccine and antibiotics. Both are essential to dealing with anthrax, but both have limitations. The anthrax vaccine takes several weeks following the first doses before immunity is initially established. The vaccine also requires multiple injections over a period of eighteen months, in addition to annual boosters, to maintain its protective effect. Antibiotics are effective in killing anthrax bacteria, but are not effective against the anthrax toxins once those toxins have been released into the blood. Antibiotics also may not be effective against antibiotic-resistant strains of anthrax.

In ABthrax, Human Genome Sciences has discovered a third critical defense against anthrax infections. In contrast to the anthrax vaccine, a single dose of ABthrax confers protection immediately following the rapid achievement of appropriate blood levels of the antibody. In contrast to antibiotics, ABthrax is effective against the lethal toxins released by anthrax bacteria. It may also prevent and treat infections by antibiotic-resistant strains of anthrax.

Results from preclinical studies conducted to date demonstrate that a single dose of ABthrax administered prophylactically or therapeutically increases survival significantly in both rabbits and nonhuman primates exposed by inhaling many times the lethal dose of anthrax

- 4 -

spores. In both models, we observed an absence of bacteria in the blood of all ABthrax-treated animals that survived. The rabbit and nonhuman primate models of inhalation anthrax are regarded as sufficient to demonstrate the efficacy of therapeutic and prophylactic agents in treating or preventing anthrax infection. A single dose of ABthrax also fully protected rats against a lethal challenge with the anthrax toxins.

Based on our preclinical results to date, we believe that ABthrax has the potential to be used both prophylactically and therapeutically. For example, ABthrax may be used to protect rescuers entering a contaminated building, soldiers in an infected environment, or exposed individuals after an attack. In addition, post-exposure treatment may lessen the natural progression of anthrax infection and increase survival. Human Genome Sciences has an Investigational New Drug application and has performed an initial Phase 1 clinical trial to evaluate the safety, tolerability, and pharmacology of ABthrax in healthy adults.

Procurement of ABthrax under Project Bioshield

Many companies have the capability and are willing to develop new products to protect against attack by biological and chemical weapons or other dangerous pathogens. A few firms, such as Human Genome Sciences, have already done so. In fact, Human Genome Sciences is among the largest and most qualified companies to participate in Project Bioshield to date. Should Human Genome Sciences prove successful in negotiating a viable business relationship with the federal government to purchase of ABthrax, it will send an extremely powerful, positive signal to similarly qualified companies to enter this market. Of course, failure by Human Genome Sciences in this endeavor could have a negative effect on the goal of stimulating greater interest of large bio-pharma companies.

The primary challenge of bio-pharma companies such as Human Genome Sciences is the absence of a commercial market for such drugs. In most cases, the only viable market is the federal government and, potentially, our foreign allies. Project Bioshield, which aims to harness public and private resources in an innovative effort to develop defenses against bioterrorism, is specifically intended to create such a market. While the Department of Health and Human Services (HHS) has always had the authority to purchase and stockpile drugs such as ABthrax outside of Project Bioshield, the statute was intended to enhance that authority. It is important to examine the first actions HHS has taken under the Project Bioshield to understand the challenges in implementing the statute, as well as the need for additional procurement reforms.

On October 26, 2004, HHS' Office of Research and Development Coordination received the first proposals to provide therapeutic products for treatment of inhalational anthrax disease in response to Solicitation No. 2004-N-01385 (the "Anthrax Therapeutics Solicitation") under what was the first, true, Project Bioshield procurement. Human Genome Sciences responded to this request with a proposal to supply ABthrax to the government.

As the first Bioshield procurement, the Anthrax Therapeutics Solicitation seeks the acquisition and maintenance within the SNS of therapeutic products to treat US civilians who have inhalational anthrax disease. The Anthrax Therapeutics Solicitation contemplates that the awarded contract(s) will be for 10 grams of an investigational new drug ("IND") final drug product ("FDP"), for use in testing, and for support for this testing. The actual manufacture of anthrax therapeutic product is an optional contract line item, which the government may decide to exercise within 12 months from the date of contract award and after the government reviews and approves IND FDP testing. While this procurement could have utilized the streamlined procurement provisions provided under Project Bioshield, the solicitation includes numerous provisions of the Federal Acquisition Regulation ("FAR") and other detailed requirements for bidders, including detailed rules governing the methods of preparing pricing for the proposal.

This initial Bioshield solicitation was curious in three ways. First, the way the solicitation structures the options in the contract fall far short of the Congressional intent of the Act to provide for a commitment to recommend funding for production for the SNS as contemplated by Project Bioshield. Contrary to the expressed intent of the Act, HHS has not committed to recommend exercise of the options for production quantities of the countermeasure upon successful development of the countermeasure. Rather, the solicitation requires bidders to propose pricing for a broad range of quantities ranging from 10,000 doses to 200,000 doses. It now appears that even if HHS awards this contract and eventually exercises its option to purchase the countermeasure, HHS is unlikely to purchase the full 200,000 doses originally proposed. This is particularly frustrating since the manufacture of this compound requires significant manufacturing startup costs. In other words, the cost per dose of 200,000 doses is significantly less than the cost per dose of 100,000 doses.

Setting a firm commitment for the quantities to be purchased, as was clearly intended by Bioshield, is critical to advance the Act's purpose of promoting the development of a biodefense industry by informing the markets that there is some certainty that there will be a government market for the product. Also, as noted above, the solicitation failed to use the simplified acquisition authorities that Bioshield makes available to the government, which would have permitted far fewer bidding requirements. As a result, this procurement process, which formally began on April 1, 2004, and has yet to be completed fourteen months later, is simply too long and too burdensome to sustain continued interest in participating in Bioshield by companies such as Human Genome Sciences whose principal focus is not the federal sector. No amount of federal appropriations can make up for the time lost in the delay in getting this contract finalized, thus costing the Nation the ability of having an Anthrax therapeutic in the stockpile until 2006, at the earliest.

Finally, HHS has caused additional uncertainty by, again inexplicably, issuing another request for information for the identical requirement, i.e., anthrax therapeutics, in the midst of the yet-to-be completed first procurement for this process. This leaves companies that responded to the first solicitation left wondering what, exactly, is the government's requirement – that is, what is the size of market, and significantly reduces the opportunity for economies of scale in the manufacture of this therapeutic. This is the very concern Project Bioshield was meant to address.

Proposed Implementation Improvements

HHS can take several steps to implement Bioshield to increase industry participation. To realize fully the legislative intent of the law, HHS should enact regulations required under the Project Bioshield Act that take into account the following issues:

- Specify that Project Bioshield Act procurements include only those FAR clauses specifically required by FAR Part 13, Simplified Acquisition Procedures;

- Provide for determinations of the order in which the government plans to procure countermeasures;

- Require HHS to specify a firm number of doses or courses of treatment in the call for countermeasures stage; and

- Provide for industry participation in market surveys undertaken during the assessment of the availability and appropriateness of countermeasures stage.

Also, as required by Section 319F-2(c)(4)(C)(ii) of the Public Health Act, HHS should, in a call for bio-terrorism countermeasures, provide industry with an estimate of the quantities of a countermeasure (in the form of number of doses or number of effective courses of treatment) that HHS intends to procure upon development of a countermeasure that meets the statutory criteria. Providing industry with wide ranges of potential requirements for a countermeasure, as HHS did in the Anthrax Therapeutics Solicitation, does not serve the statutory purpose of promoting the development of a biodefense industry because it introduces additional uncertainty about the size of the government market for the countermeasure.

HHS and the Department of Homeland Security ("DHS") should provide industry with information concerning the implementation of the Project Bioshield Act. For example, HHS and DHS should provide industry and the public with a status report concerning the governmental processes required by Section 319F-2(c)(2)-(6) of the Public Health Act.

Perhaps most importantly, DHS should inform industry of the progress and priority of the required threat assessments so that companies can make proper business decisions in their planning process. Project Bioshield requires that the DHS, in conjunction with the HHS, conduct a threat assessment to "assess current and emerging threats of chemical, biological radiological, and nuclear agents; and determine which of such agents present a material threat against the United States population sufficient to affect national security" and for which a countermeasure is needed. As implemented, this threat assessment must be conducted prior to any decision to purchase a needed countermeasure under the Project Bioshield.

In addition to the specific recommendations above that should be taken into account during the regulatory process and in order to carry forth the initiative's legislative intent, we have several policy suggestions that should be considered in implementing Project Bioshield:

First and foremost, HHS should make clear that the statute does not require contractors to comply with burdensome government procurement requirements, including the requirement for certified cost and pricing data, in order to stimulate the maximum interest possible by commercial companies. Similarly, HHS should avoid the use of cost-type contracts or contract line items (thus, eliminating the need for a proposed contractor to adopt non-GAAP accounting practices) wherever possible.

HHS should structure Bioshield contracts to avoid a "staged" procurement approach such as that announced in the recent Anthrax therapeutic request for proposal, wherever possible. While we recognize the need for staged procurements under certain circumstances, using this method where HHS has conducted proper market research will avoid unnecessary delays and unpredictable results, thereby stimulating far greater private sector interest.

Timing is critical. Agencies responsible for administering Project Bioshield should take a proactive approach to identifying, evaluating and procuring effective drugs. I applaud the Subcommittee for its continued oversight of this critical bio-defense program. Near-term delays in evaluating and securing the production of viable countermeasures can disproportionately prolong the procurement of such drugs. In the case of ABthrax, Human Genome Sciences is ready to move the drug into production, which will require significant investment to secure a manufacturing facility and perfect the manufacturing process. Due to the demand for such specialized facilities, a delay of months now could postpone delivery of the drug by over a year. We are also ready to begin advanced clinical safety trials in humans, having already demonstrated the drug's efficacy in animals and initial safety in humans. To date, ABthrax has been developed entirely with private funds, but in order to move forward the company needs a commitment from the federal government to develop, manufacture and purchase the drug. With sufficient government support, Human Genome Sciences can begin producing significant quantities of ABthrax by the end of next year. We look forward to formalizing this commitment in a contract with HHS in the coming weeks and appreciate every effort to ensure the maximum quantities of ABthrax are purchased for the stockpile as soon as possible without any further delay.

Thank you again for this opportunity to testify and I look forward to answering your questions.

Mr. MARCHANT. Thank you, Dr. Davis.

The Chair recognizes Chairman Shays.

Mr. SHAYS. Gentlemen, thank you for being here today. I feel badly that I could not ask some questions of the previous panel because I wanted to get into the stovepiping and so on. I wanted to get into why DOD has one program and others have another and I wanted to get into the connection between them.

What did you hear from the previous panel that you agreed with the most and that you would disagree with the most? I would ask that of each of you. Dr. Hanna.

Dr. HANNA. I agreed with the statement made by HHS representatives that working with large pharmaceutical companies is not really going to work. They really could make much more money with a cardiovascular drug than they can with these types of vaccines. There are many vaccines that were made that were never used because they couldn't make any money selling them. The countries that were going to use them couldn't afford to pay for them.

Working with the smaller, mid-size, biotechnology companies is probably clearly the way to go. Unfortunately, even those companies are not going to do some of this work on contracts or grants because they can't make a living at a 6 percent margin on the work they do but this is the way the legislation is written to allow them to fund their programs.

I think the legislation needs to be changed to allow for multiple awards, grants or contracts or allow companies to come in and do it on their own but still let them compete. This is the way good science gets done in the major projects this country has launched.

Mr. SHAYS. What statement did you disagree with the most by any of the previous panelists?

Dr. HANNA. I disagreed with the fact that the vaccines in the JVAP Program and in some of the other programs are difficult to accomplish. We could have had an anthrax vaccine a couple of years ago, we could have had a couple hundred thousand botulinum antitoxin, polyclonal equine botulinum antitoxin in our repertoire. The urgency is there at the top level at the present and it is at the congressional level and the Senate level and at the top offices of these departments but when it filters down to the functionaries, the urgency is lost and the status quo steps in and this is demotivating to the small, medium or large pharmaceutical companies.

Mr. SHAYS. Explain to me why we don't have progress in those two areas? Tell me specifically why. You are saying it is motivate up here but what specifically wasn't done that should have been done?

Dr. HANNA. It is my understanding that the legislation doesn't allow them to think outside the envelope, that they have to function according to the legislation and the legislation allows them to award a contract to the lowest bidder and that contract is what they live with. If they would allow them to award several contracts simultaneously for the same project and let them compete to Phase 1 trials and the one that gets to the Phase 1 trials and can work with the FDA the fastest ends up with the purchase order is the way to go.

Mr. SHAYS. You are saying that you would cover the research costs for the three or four that would get involved?

Dr. HANNA. We offered to do it through private investment. We had investors.

Mr. SHAYS. You were willing to compete privately in a contest because you believe you would have had a better product in the end?

Dr. HANNA. We have already made it, we had already made it. We spent $25 million of DOD's money to make the first 5,000.

Mr. SHAYS. I know that and that is why I am asking you why we don't have it? What in the law prevented them from moving forward with you?

Dr. HANNA. I don't know. I spoke to somebody recently who is well known in this area and he said the law just prohibits a multiple contract or multiple awards for the same project.

Mr. SHAYS. Why would they have had to do multiple awards? If you already had it, why couldn't they just contract to you?

Dr. HANNA. They did. They contracted a foreign company. HHS contracted a foreign company to make it.

Mr. SHAYS. Because you were a higher bidder? You weren't the lower bidder?

Dr. HANNA. We didn't bid at all.

Mr. SHAYS. Why?

Dr. HANNA. We were offering to do it at our own costs.

Mr. SHAYS. You are confusing me. This has not been a great day, so maybe it is my problem but be patient with me here. You had a product that DOD helped you develop?

Dr. HANNA. They contracted with us to develop, yes.

Mr. SHAYS. They gave you money to develop the product. You developed the product. Are they saying the product won't do the job?

Dr. HANNA. No.

Mr. SHAYS. Are they saying the product costs too much money?

Dr. HANNA. No. The project ended in 1997 and there was no urgency and need for it.

Mr. SHAYS. But the project ended then but you still had the capability to produce the product?

Dr. HANNA. We have had the capability from 1997 to now.

Mr. SHAYS. So why do you want me to be so confused here?

Dr. HANNA. I am not trying to.

Mr. SHAYS. There has to be a reason.

Dr. HANNA. I don't have an answer. I can think of no reason. I thought there had to be a reason also.

Mr. SHAYS. This is a conversation we had somewhat privately and I thought you would be able to publicly put on the record.

Dr. HANNA. I did at the suggestion of NIAID, Tony Fauci's group, I did put in at their request an unsolicited proposal to the CDC to make this product and it was rejected.

Mr. SHAYS. Did they give you a reason why?

Dr. HANNA. No, but they turned around and awarded the contract to this foreign company which we heard today was having extreme difficulties getting geared up to make the product.

Mr. SHAYS. Dr. Davis, can you enlighten me about this issue?

Dr. DAVIS. I am not sure I can enlighten you about his issue, no. We have been facing a slightly different issue in that the Government clearly appears to have some interest in our product, it has been a long procurement process and as a consequence, our concern is that the delay makes it very difficult for us to plan and makes it very difficult for us and other companies to be willing to develop from their own funds products. There is a need for different procurement methods for different things. There are clearly some products where the Federal Government probably needs to fund the early research in order to get it done but there are also other products and other capabilities like ours where we have done the vast majority of the research and the development on our own. What we need is a commitment from the Government to buy the product and we need a commitment to buy it in sufficient quantities frankly to make it worthwhile. If somebody only wants a few thousand doses, we are not going to start a large scale manufacturing facility and dedicate 3 to 4 months of manufacturing capability to make a few thousand doses. If they want 100,000 doses, that starts to get economically reasonable. If they want 200,000 doses, it makes a lot of sense. For us to go into future products or other companies like us to go into future products, you need to state up front what is really the need of the Government. They have told us they want an anthrax antibody but never told us how many doses they really want, never told us what schedule they really want it on and so we are left in a quandary of how we develop this product. We have other pharmaceutical products competing.

Mr. SHAYS. Do you think they have told other companies what they want?

Dr. DAVIS. No, no. I don't think they are being disingenuous here, I think they are in a quandary about what they want or maybe they know and haven't specified. The RFP asks us to bid on prices for doses between 10,000 doses and 200,000 doses. That is a tremendous difference in how you manufacture.

Mr. SHAYS. So you give them a bid at 10,000 and a bid at 50,000, a bid at 100,000, a bid at 15,000.

Dr. DAVIS. That is exactly what we have done.

Mr. SHAYS. So what is difficult about that?

Dr. DAVIS. The problem is that the manufacturing needs to be planned 12 to 18 months ahead of time.

Mr. SHAYS. That is another issue but the bidding issue isn't there.

Dr. DAVIS. No, we can bid. It's very difficult to know, however, if you see that RFP and they are really only thinking about 10,000 doses, we may not want to play. It is simply not enough economic incentive even if we charge astronomical amounts for 10,000 doses.

Mr. SHAYS. Is it that difficult to do a bid response? In other words, you price the 10,000 at such an extreme price that you are not in the running but you give them a price?

Dr. DAVIS. And we have done that.

Mr. SHAYS. So that is not really the issue. With all due respect, that is not the issue.

Dr. DAVIS. It is an issue in terms of are we going to go after another project like this, are we going to use our own money to do the research and development on another project if we are not sure what the Government needs?

Mr. SHAYS. Let me ask you, do you do the research before you do the bid or do you do the bid before you do the research?

Dr. DAVIS. In this case, we did the research before the bid because we thought there would be a market. I think in the future, we are unlikely to do anything more in this area without a clear indication of what they want in terms of quantities.

Mr. SHAYS. What is the statement you agreed with most and the statement you disagreed with the most and who made that statement?

Dr. DAVIS. Dr. Fauci I think made the statement that I agree with the most that this does have to be a partnership between the Government and industry. The Government does not have the capability to do large scale manufacture of these products. It is very expensive, takes very specialized facilities but we do need a partner in the Government so we know what we are doing and when they want it and what it is.

I think it is hard to say there is a single statement I disagree with. I think I am concerned that the procurement process for the BioShield as described is not going as smoothly as some may think. I think it still has a lot of work to be done to make it more efficient, there are a lot of contract provisions, a lot of indemnity and liability issues that are a hurdle for companies to be willing to go across in order to enter this market.

Mr. SHAYS. Thank you.

Mr. MARCHANT. I have a couple questions and they will be questions broached from a freshman in the Congress, just a couple of elementary questions.

If the Government came to you tomorrow and said we want 200,000 doses of this, how long would it take you to produce them?

Dr. DAVIS. We would be able to start production in approximately 12 to 18 months, but it would take us probably 6 months, maybe a year to produce all those doses but they would be in a rolling batch. We could have doses available. For example, if they told us today they wanted 200,000 doses, we could certainly have doses for them at the beginning of 2007 and all the doses by the end of 2007.

Mr. MARCHANT. How much public knowledge would be available about the amount of doses and the antibody that was being produced?

Dr. DAVIS. I would presume, and speak with a little ignorance here, that the contract would be public and the number of doses they requested would be specified. The precise structure of the antibody and the nature of the antibody we have been fairly careful not to make public for security reasons but some of that would depend on the Government's desire to keep it secret or not.

Mr. MARCHANT. From someone that thinks the Government or some entity has an antibody for any of these diseases can be introduced in any form in the water system, through milk, etc., do you feel the American citizen has a security that there are vaccines, antibodies and things available immediately that can be introduced that can combat these things or are they aware that we are studying this?

Dr. DAVIS. I think it depends on the particular agent you are talking about and the particular means of which the product is distributed and how you can treat it. In many cases, there are inadequate therapies today. In some cases, there are some therapies which may be adequate in some circumstances and not in others.

Mr. MARCHANT. Obviously the general knowledge of the cure will make sure whatever entity decides to introduce this into society will not introduce that?

Dr. DAVIS. There is a strong deterrent effect one would think from having stockpile of an efficient deterrent.

Dr. HANNA. The best offense is a good defense in this case, clearly.

Mr. MARCHANT. So if DOD or whatever entity decided they needed to have sufficient vaccine on hand to combat, how prepared are we at this moment for those diseases that could be introduced?

Dr. HANNA. You are not. For most of them, you are not prepared.

Mr. MARCHANT. You in your case were paid to develop one but you were not paid to produce the doses?

Dr. HANNA. Let me try to clarify one thing. When we stopped making it, we closed down our manufacturing facility. We recognize one of the problems and why we might have been discriminated against is because our manufacturing facility didn't exist, so we went back and said, we will volunteer with private funds to build that manufacturing facility again and within 18 months we will deliver to you 50,000 doses that meet the specs, that would be FDA-approved again as we did previously for emergency use and we would get it fully licensed eventually.

I think at that time, they decided it would be better to go to another contractor that had a facility and underestimated the degree of scientific capability required because you heard Simonson say that it is not only science, there is a bit of an art to it and it is, there is an art to it. It is not something that everybody can do. This contractor is working very hard, I am sure, but they are not able to accomplish it yet. They will eventually.

Mr. MARCHANT. They own the formula?

Dr. HANNA. We have the patent on the procedure.

Mr. MARCHANT. So they have to deal with you?

Dr. HANNA. We have not discussed that with them but my point is it would have been better, it would have been smarter to let them go and have the security of the contract they managed and release us with a commitment that if we did what we said, they would purchase from us at a fair price. Then you would have had both competing with each other. That would have been the smartest way to do it. Instead, they went the contract route, which is the one they know the best.

All I am saying is we need to start some competition however we do it, whether we do it with multiple contracts, a contract versus an independent operation, with a commitment letter. We couldn't raise the money without the commitment letter. All we wanted was a letter saying if you do it, we will buy it at a fair price to be negotiated.

Mr. MARCHANT. Mr. Counsel. Chairman Shays.

Mr. SHAYS. If you both were running the program, how would you run the program? When I say program, we have agricultural needs, we have plant needs, animal needs, we have human needs, so it makes sense you would have three separate tracks, correct, for each of those?

Dr. HANNA. Yes.

Mr. SHAYS. How would you run the program differently? If you were in charge of this program, suppose the United States says, I want you to run this program, tell me how you are going to run it, what would you say?

Dr. HANNA. I would do it basically as I described. Let us deal first with the biological. We know what the agents are. Smallpox is pretty well covered, we have plenty of vaccine for smallpox. What we don't have is vaccine for the other nine agents or some kind of a therapeutic.

Mr. SHAYS. When you say agent versus therapeutic, with anthrax there is one element that prevents it from catching hold and another is you have it and now how you deal with it. Is that your difference when you talk about agent versus therapeutic?

Dr. HANNA. I am talking about a vaccine that would protect you versus a therapeutic that you would take after you had contact and in some cases, there will be no vaccines. The botulism vaccine they were talking about was AB. Those are the two common forms. If anyone was going to use an agent, it wouldn't be AB. That is the most common and they know that. They would use C through G and those are the most difficult to defend against.

I would rank them and I would do just what I said. I would set up multiple awards. I would either allow companies to come in and give them commitment letters that if they do it, we will purchase it or I would set up a contract and an award at the same time. I would do what we do in the pharmaceutical industry. Oftentimes, when new projects are started, we set up two, maybe three groups and let them compete.

Mr. SHAYS. That sounds more expensive to me.

Dr. HANNA. It is a lot more expensive to go with the low bitter and come up 7, 8 or 9 years later with the vaccines we have seen from JVAP.

Mr. SHAYS. You are saying, get more companies and individuals involved, you will get a product sooner, it is going to cost you more, but we won't be where we are now with nothing?

Dr. HANNA. How do you compare the cost when you have a situation where you have nothing and still the threat is equal to what it was 5 years ago?

Mr. SHAYS. What I am hearing you say in a sense is that by doing it this way, it is taking longer which means we remain vulnerable when we don't have to remain vulnerable. Your view would be that we would get there sooner with a better product if we had multiple competition?

Dr. HANNA. And build in redundancies. That is the thing missing here, redundancies. You have a JVAP program with no redundancies backing it. The one redundancy for the anthrax vaccine, they can't even award it yet. This would be a redundancy to what is in the JVAP program. You can't get them to make a decision. I think the problem is the legislation is written to favor the status quo which is to do it through grants and contracts, and grants and contracts allow you to give a contract for a particular project. I am saying set up competition.

In NASA, they had a redundancy for everything, everything had a backup. That is how they got to the moon and got back but that was a Presidential mandate that said make it happen. We are doing it in the standard way and I think we have to start thinking out of the envelope.

Mr. SHAYS. I hear you and I understand now what you were trying to tell me. It finally sunk in. Thank you.

Dr. Davis.

Dr. DAVIS. I think that is main thing I would change.

Mr. SHAYS. You are running the program.

Dr. DAVIS. I am running the program. I think the way I would set it up is one, I would be very clear and they have been, these are the agents, the terrorist weapons that we are most concerned about and I would then give a clear indication of what is the amount of need for product and then I would put out an RFP but I would streamline the bureaucratic process. I would use simplified contracting methods, I would try to bring pressure to get the time lines down to much less.

Fourteen months for RFI to still have a contract negotiation is a long time and we have been waiting simply for the contract before we even begin our manufacturing. So if you can streamline that process, you will get these products on line sooner. If you have a clear, up front commitment, streamlined process, I think you will find more industry interest in participating in these sorts of programs because then you can do a real measure of the net present value of this project and understand whether it is worth your investment or not.

Mr. SHAYS. The way counsel is responding to my question to him as you were talking about what you were saying was that you would use the more traditional system but make sure there was a pot of gold and incentive.

Dr. DAVIS. Yes.

Mr. SHAYS. You would have an incentive but you would have a competitive process and both of you would deal with speeding up the time process?

Dr. HANNA. Of course.

Dr. DAVIS. Yes.

Mr. SHAYS. When you heard what was said today, is your emotion just disappointment, disgust? The reason I am asking is I am trying to figure out how I should feel about this. Is it just give me a break or is it something like, you know what, this is going to happen, we are vulnerable and you guys are at fault in the end. Tell me what level of feeling you have right now.

Dr. HANNA. My level of feeling is disappointment. It has been a lot of energy. I think everybody at this table has done their darnedest to get the job done. I have known people in the agencies who came in thinking they could get the job done and then ran into so many obstacles that they ended up leaving.

We walked away from it and decided we are not going to get involved and do this thing because we couldn't, we couldn't get it done. So it is disappointment. I think the disappointment is that while there was an urgency and while there was a concern, we didn't come up with enough creative mechanisms to get the job done and we allowed each agency to funnel through their own process, muddle through their own process individually. This is an interdisciplinary need. You need a lot of people to get this job done. You need industry, you need the Government agencies, and you need people who are highly motivated and have a reason for being motivated.

I would say disappointment and encouragement that looking forward that you had this hearing and maybe we will get something done and something will come out of it.

Mr. SHAYS. Let me say in regards to that, we may end up having a private meeting with the folks I didn't get to question but we know we need to do something different and we need to move this along more quickly.

Dr. Davis, your emotion?

Dr. DAVIS. I think my emotion continues to be a certain amount of frustration. I believe the agencies are very dedicated to getting this done. I think their hearts and their minds are in the right place. I think they have not been able to motivate the bureaucracy to move and we need to find a way to make this a more efficient process. Otherwise, you are going to end up with more companies like mine who are frustrated and simply aren't going to play.

Mr. SHAYS. Thank you, Mr. Chairman. Thank you both very much.

Mr. MARCHANT. The subcommittee is adjourned.

[Whereupon, at 3:59 p.m., the subcommittee was adjourned.]

[The prepared statements of Hon. Dennis J. Kucinich, Hon. C.A. Dutch Ruppersberger, and Hon. Bernard Sanders follow:]

Statement of Rep. Dennis Kucinich
Ranking Minority Member
House Subcommittee on National Security, Emerging
Threats and International Relations
Committee on Government Reform
U.S. House of Representatives

Hearing on "Elusive Antidotes: Progress Developing
Chemical Biological Radiological and Nuclear (CBRN)
Countermeasures"

June 14, 2005

Thank you for holding this hearing Mr. Chairman, and thank

you to all of the experts here before the Subcommittee today. I

believe it is incredibly important for us all to be in the same room

together, for today we are literally discussing saving lives.

The United States has the foremost scientific laboratories and

one of the most advanced drug research and development

structures in the world. We know more about infectious diseases

now than at any point in history. Yet, in spite of all of this, we are

all still extremely vulnerable to just a few microscopic spores of anthrax, or dozens of other deadly pathogens through food, water, air, animals and people.

I remember when Congress was shut down in 2001 and 2002 because mail containing anthrax spores was sent here. I recall the protective gear my staff needed to wear just to open letters from our constituents, and the escape hood masks we've all been trained to wear in an emergency. We all felt helpless and vulnerable. I would hope our preparedness for a similar threat has improved since then, but I'm not so sure it has.

It disturbs me that since the 2001 anthrax attacks on Congress, we have had little or no supply of anthrax vaccine in the Strategic National Stockpile. It concerns me that other agencies, as well as the drug manufacturers who will produce these countermeasures, are not getting the guidance they need from DHS, who I understand will not finish their comprehensive threat assessment of the highest priority toxic agents until the end of 2006.

In addition, we also need to open up the deliberative process. In May, five million doses of an established anthrax vaccine were ordered by DHS and HHS for the Stockpile, yet we weren't told why only this small number was requested, given that it is a multiple dose regime.

In 2003, $1.5 billion was spent on developing a smallpox vaccine, but nobody could quantify what the threat was. How do we know that it made sense to spend that money? Was the threat of smallpox more urgent than that of preparing for a flu pandemic? Was the threat sufficient to take that $1.5 billion away from funding for HIV/AIDS research or education programs or Social Security? Or are scarce budget resources being spent only on what William Raub, the HHS Deputy Assistant Secretary for Public Health Emergency Preparedness admitted last week was "low hanging fruit" – where a substantial research base is already present.

I know each of the agencies are doing the best it can, and that fighting both Mother Nature and terrorists at the same time are formidable tasks – we must not fight amongst ourselves too.

Rather, we must stay ahead of the curve, and work together to fund the best science and technology that exists in order to solve these problems. It is vital that we stay proactive and anticipate future CBRN threats, not just merely respond to them.

Thank you, Mr. Chairman, and I look forward to listening to the testimony of the witnesses today.

Congressman C.A. Dutch Ruppersberger
Subcommittee on National Security, Emerging Threats, and
International Relations

**"Elusive Antidotes: Progress Developing Chemical Biological
Radiological and Nuclear (CBRN) Countermeasures"**

June 14, 2005

Statement:

Thank you Mr. Chairman for holding this subcommittee hearing

regarding the National Security, Emerging Threats, and

International Relations to examine federal efforts to develop

medical countermeasures for Chemical Biological Radiological

and Nuclear (CBRN) agents.

My major concern that I have with this hearing is "Are we

preparing for the correct attack?" "What else is out there that we

are not focusing on?" Biological weapons have been a problem for

society ever since their first recorded use in the sixth century B.C.

Despite the recent media infatuation with bioterrorism and its sibling, bio warfare, we're not exactly talking about a new idea here, either globally or in the United States instead I want to know what Congress can do or what we need to know in order to prepare ourselves and the American people for another attack.

I am also concerned about the misuse of Anthrax. I believe that if people stockpile antibiotics on their own, there may be shortages for those who need the medication. This could also result in inappropriate use of antibiotics, an important factor in the emergence of drug-resistant germs.

According to, The Baltimore Sun, in a push to control their own fate, Montgomery County, Baltimore City and other jurisdictions around the country are spending federal homeland security grant money to create stockpiles of antidotes that duplicate drugs readily available through the six-year-old Strategic National Stockpile program, which has cost more than $2 billion to assemble.

In Baltimore City and Montgomery County alone, the cost for drugs has totaled about $100,000 since the terrorist and anthrax attacks of 2001. In surveys taken by the Baltimore City Health Department, emergency personnel said fear for the safety of their families would be a deterrent to responding immediately to a biological attack. That survey concerns me as we continue to learn about new attacks and groups that threaten our well being. Sure, we are stockpiling anthrax, but what about the other biological agents that take aim at threatening this countries livelihood. A bioterrorist attack in my opinion will not be white powder floating out of the sky. It will be something obvious and that something obvious is what concerns me the most.

As we continue to discuss how to best examine the efficiency and effectiveness of countermeasures among government defense and health agencies I hope to be given a clear understanding of where we are in terms of these major threats. Being exposed to chemical or biological warfare agents is not something that I take lightly when it comes to our men and woman serving our nation. It disturbs me that as a power nation we still do not have all the needed vaccines against Chemical Biological Radiological and Nuclear agents when it comes to our service members or the general public. We need to look at the wider spectrum here and be clear at what and who we are looking for. My concern and commitment will always be the welfare of this nation.

I look forward to hearing the testimony presented today and I look forward to asking questions of the witnesses.

Thank You.

STATEMENT BY REP. BERNARD SANDERS BEFORE THE NATIONAL SECURITY SUBCOMMITTEE HEARING ON CHEMICAL, BIOLOGICAL, RADIOLOGICAL, AND NUCLEAR COUNTERMEASURES ON TUESDAY, JUNE 14, 2005 AT 2:00PM IN 2154 RAYBURN

Chairman Shays and Ranking Member Kucinich, thank you for holding this important hearing. I would also like to welcome our witnesses for being with us today.

It is critical that this Subcommittee take a serious look at the progress being made by the federal government to develop medical countermeasures to protect our military and our citizens against Chemical, Biological, Radiological, and Nuclear (CBRN) agents.

Mr. Chairman, as you know full well, the Persian Gulf War of 1990-1991, reminded all of us of how susceptible we are to chemical and biological warfare. While 700,000 Americans participated in the Gulf War, incredibly, some 100,000 of those soldiers eventually became ill with a myriad of symptoms which have been referred to as Gulf War Illness. Mr. Chairman, I have been proud to work with you over the past decade on this issue, and I look forward to continuing our efforts towards finding a cure for this illness which has caused so much pain to our veterans and their family members.

If we are going to reduce the vulnerability to a terrorist CBRN attack which we must, we have got to have a firm grasp of what caused Gulf War Illness and how it can be effectively treated.

And, Mr. Chairman, in the 1950s, thousands of American soldiers became ill with cancer and other diseases because of exposure to nuclear radiation at A-bomb testing sites.

But, our soldiers are not the only ones susceptible to CBRN threats.

All of us remember that in 2001, deadly anthrax spores were distributed through our own postal system targeted at members of the news media, and Members of Congress.

And, today, according to U.S. intelligence officials, it is believed that al Qaeda and other terrorist groups are pursuing the production of mustard agents, sarin gas, and so-called "dirty bombs."

Given these developments it is absolutely imperative that we develop strong medical countermeasures to protect the public against these deadly agents.

But, since the 2001 anthrax attacks, we still do not have an adequate supply of anthrax vaccine in the Strategic National Stockpile. That is something we must address.

In addition, in 2003, $1.5 billion was spent on developing a smallpox vaccine, but nobody could quantify what the threat was. How do we know that it made sense to spend that money? Was the threat of smallpox more urgent than that of preparing for a flu epidemic for example?

Mr. Chairman, we have the greatest public health system in the world. We know more about infectious diseases now than at any point in history. But, in spite of all of this, we must not forget that we are still extremely vulnerable to just a few spores of anthrax or dozens of other deadly viruses passed and spread from the food we eat, the water we drink, or the air we breathe.

That is why it is crucial that we stay ahead of the curve and work together to fund the best science and technology that exists in order to solve these problems. We must be proactive and anticipate future threats, not just merely respond to them.

This is not an academic exercise. The discussion we are holding today is literally about saving lives. Mr. Chairman, thank you again for holding this hearing. And, I look forward to hearing from our witnesses.

○